EVALUATION AND TREATMENT OF POSTPARTUM EMOTIONAL DISORDERS

Ann L. Dunnewold, PhD

Independent Practice
Dallas, Texas
President of Postpartum Support International
(1996-1998)

Professional Resource Press
Sarasota, Florida

Published by
Professional Resource Press
(An imprint of the Professional Resource Exchange, Inc.)
Post Office Box 15560
Sarasota, FL 34277-1560

Printed in the United States of America

The copy editor was Brian Fogarty, the managing editor was Debra Fink, the production coordinator was Laurie Girsch, and the cover designer was Bill Tabler.

Library of Congress Cataloging-in-Publication Data

Dunnewold, Ann.
    Evaluation and treatment of postpartum emotional disorders / Ann
L. Dunnewold.
        p.   cm. -- (Practitioner's resource series)
    Includes bibliographical references.
    ISBN 1-56887-024-8 (pbk. : alk. paper)
    1. Postpartum psychiatric disorders. I. Title II. Series.
RG850.D86 1996
618.7'6--DC21   96-47166
                                                         CIP

PREFACE TO THE SERIES

As a publisher of books, cassettes, and continuing education programs, the Professional Resource Press and Professional Resource Exchange, Inc. strive to provide mental health professionals with highly applied resources that can be used to enhance clinical skills and expand practical knowledge.

All titles in the *Practitioner's Resource Series* are designed to provide important new information on topics of vital concern to psychologists, clinical social workers, marriage and family therapists, psychiatrists, and other mental health professionals.

Although the focus and content of each book in this series will be quite different, there will be notable similarities:

1. Each title in the series will address a timely topic of critical clinical importance.

2. The target audience for each title will be practicing mental health professionals. Our authors were chosen for their ability to provide concrete "how-to-do-it" guidance to colleagues who are trying to increase their competence in dealing with complex clinical problems.

3. The information provided in these books will represent "state-of-the-art" information and techniques derived from both clinical experience and empirical research. Each of these guide books will include references and resources

for those who wish to pursue more advanced study of the discussed topic.

4. The authors will provide numerous case studies, specific recommendations for practice, and the types of "nitty-gritty" details that clinicians need before they can incorporate new concepts and procedures into their practices.

We feel that one of the unique assets of the Professional Resource Press is that all of its editorial decisions are made by mental health professionals. The publisher, all editorial consultants, and all reviewers are practicing psychologists, marriage and family therapists, clinical social workers, and psychiatrists.

If there are other topics you would like to see addressed in this series, please let me know.

Lawrence G. Ritt, Publisher

ABSTRACT

As mental health professionals have studied postpartum depression, they have determined that there is no one discrete entity, but rather a variety of syndromes and symptoms which affect a woman after the birth of a baby. This has lead to the broader concept of postpartum emotional disorders, which encompasses the full range of emotional health related to childbirth. These postpartum emotional disorders, ranging from mild depression and anxiety to panic, mania, and psychosis, affect at least 40,000 women a year.

While interest in postpartum emotional disorders lapsed in the U.S. after the American Psychiatric Association removed the concept from the first *Diagnostic and Statistical Manual of Mental Disorders (DSM)*, recent interest and research has increased, as professionals begin to recognize these many syndromes and the large numbers of women who are affected. For many women, depression and anxiety arising after the birth of a baby represent the first contact with the mental health system. Misunderstanding and misinformation persist among health and mental health professionals alike about what many women experience after the birth of a baby and how to intervene effectively. In this volume, a careful review of the research illuminates the current state of knowledge about these disorders. Guidelines are presented for assessment of these clients and their families, and case studies illustrate the many ways in which postpartum emotional problems go beyond depression. Concrete, effective treatment ideas are presented, so that professionals can offer empathetic, informed help for this life transition and make this first contact with the mental health system a positive and productive experience.

TABLE OF CONTENTS

DIAGNOSIS AND TREATMENT *(Continued)*

EVALUATION AND TREATMENT OF POSTPARTUM EMOTIONAL DISORDERS

ETIOLOGY

HISTORY OF RECOGNIZING AND TREATING POSTPARTUM DISORDERS: THE IMPETUS FOR CHANGE

Postpartum psychiatric illness was first described by Hippocrates in the fourth century BC. In the 19th century, Marcé, a French physician, noted the close connection between the known physical changes of the puerperium and the appearance of symptoms such as confusion and delirium (Hamilton, 1992). In the early 20th century this connection was obscured as the psychiatric community explored the etiology of mental illness, developing a nomenclature to reflect each condition's cause (Hamilton, 1992). Most of the then-known psychiatric illnesses fit neatly into three broad categories: dementia praecox (later to be called schizophrenia), manic and depressive (affective) reactions, and toxic-exhaustive psychoses (later to be called organic). Postpartum emotional disorders did not fit this classification, so the term "post-partum" was discredited and eliminated, ignoring Marcé's work. This move was finalized in the development of the first edition of the official U.S. nomenclature, the *Diagnostic and Statistical Manual of Mental Disorders* (*DSM*; American Psychiatric Association [APA], 1952). Generations passed with little attention to postpartum emotions (Brockington & Cox-Roper, 1988).

Interest emerged again when R. E. Gordon and K. K. Gordon (1959) focused on less severe emotional reactions after childbirth. Large-scale studies by Brice Pitt (1968) and others in the early 1960s generated the first data on prevalence and correlates of "postpartum depression." The Marcé Society, established in 1980 to study psychiatric aspects of childbearing, fueled research interest, providing a forum for academic and clinical knowledge. With the arrival of *DSM-IV* (APA, 1994), it is possible to designate postpartum onset for a major depressive disorder, though other postpartum emotional difficulties are unrecognized in this "official" nomenclature, as well as in the most recent version of the *International Classification of Disorders* (*ICD-9*; World Health Organization, 1978).

The debate continues as to whether postpartum depression is a distinct diagnosis, with some investigators asserting that there is a biological and/or symptom pattern distinction while others argue that only timing differentiates postpartum from nonpostpartum depression (Whiffen, 1992). Ballard and colleagues (1994) studied 200 couples at 6 weeks and 6 months postpartum. Depression rates did not differ significantly between this group and the control group of parents of 3- to 5-year-old children. These researchers noted that many of their subjects scored just under the threshold of "major depression." O'Hara et al. (1990) recruited a large sample of childbearing women, matched for control purposes with an equal-sized sample of nonchildbearing women, and evaluated mood state, marital, and social adjustment. There were no differences between the two groups in major and minor rates of depression during pregnancy and the postpartum period.

Childbearing women experienced significantly higher levels of depressive symptomatology and poorer social adjustment than their nonchildbearing counterparts. Whiffen and Gotlib (1993) compared a sample ($N = 900$) of postpartum women diagnosed with depression with a nonpostpartum depressed group and two nondepressed control groups. They concluded that the typical episode of postpartum depression is mild, with 70% of the postpartum depressed women meeting criteria for minor but not major depression. Although mild and on the level of an adjustment disorder, these episodes were still evident 6 months later.

Both of these studies, while controlling many factors uncontrolled in previous research, utilized the Beck Depression Inventory (BDI; A. T. Beck et al., 1961) and the Schedule of Affective Disorders and Schizophrenia (SADS; Endicott & Spitzer, 1978) as their primary tools to assess depression. Hopkins, S. B. Campbell, and Marcus (1989) examined the course of normal postpartum adjustment compared to the symptomatology of postpartum depression, and found a lack of concordance between the BDI and the SADS interviews. They concluded that the BDI may not be an appropriate instrument for use in a postpartum sample, given its tendency to both over- and underdiagnose depression in this group. Similarly, Field and her colleagues (1991) highlighted the difficulties possible with self-report measures, the BDI in particular. They discovered that mothers diagnosed with depression who scored zero on the BDI had greater problems interacting with their infants than did women diagnosed with depression who had mean scores of 20 on the BDI.

Similarly, Affonso and colleagues (Affonso et al., 1990) conducted a longitudinal study of 202 first-time mothers using the SADS (Endicott & Spitzer, 1978) and Research Diagnostic Criteria (Spitzer, Endicott, & Robins, 1981) at four periods across pregnancy and the postpartum period. Discovering that the standard SADS interview was not sufficient to differentiate a childbearing woman's normal symptoms from those of depression, they modified the SADS, labeling the new form SADS-PPG (SADS-

3

Pregnancy and Postpartum Guidelines; Affonso et al., 1990). They tested this revision on a separate, preliminary sample of 25 women. Using the SADS-PPG protected against the false positive symptoms that can arise when normal symptoms of pregnancy and the postpartum, such as appetite or sleep disturbance, are attributed to depression in the full form of the SADS. The SADS-PPG identified low intensity symptoms of a labile, oscillating character which are common postpartum, but would otherwise be masked or go undetected. Their results indicated that misdiagnosis (i.e., false positives) of childbearing women's depressive reactions is a probability given the assumption of similarity between postpartum and nonpostpartum depression. Inaccuracy may result when research or clinical assessments are made using instruments which are not specific to the normal concerns of postpartum women.

Another artifact of the research which prevents a firm conclusion about the distinct nature of postpartum depression is the timing of assessments. Gotlib et al. (1989) point out that, in general, prevalence rates obtained later in the postpartum period are higher than those found in the first 2 weeks after delivery. In recent research, Gjerdingen and Chaloner (1994) saw that mental health was generally poorest at 4 weeks postpartum, and they continued their assessments for 12 months postpartum. Miller, Barr, and Eaton (1993) reported 6 weeks postpartum as the peak distress period for new mothers. Pop et al. (1993) discovered that women were significantly more depressed at 10 weeks postpartum than at any other time during pregnancy or postpartum. In a study of anxiety, depression, and hostility across pregnancy and the postpartum period, York et al. (1992) found that intensity of these emotions decreased across pregnancy and the early postpartum assessment at 6 weeks, only to rise to significant levels again at 3 months postpartum. Demyttenaere et al. (1995) had similar findings, with higher depression levels seen in the third trimester and at 6 months postpartum than at either 5 days or 6 weeks postpartum. If every study finds a different "peak" time for negative postpartum emotions, then consistent, controlled research to definitively answer the question of what postpartum women experience is formidable.

Finally, an answer to the question of distinct diagnosis in postpartum depression remains elusive due to a focus on depression alone. Recently, syndromes of postpartum obsessive-compulsive disorder (OCD), panic disorder, and stress reactions have been detailed in the literature (Metz, Sichel, & Goff, 1988; Moleman, Van der Hart, & Van der Kolk, 1992; Sichel et al., 1993). To date, no large-scale, controlled study of postpartum emotions has attempted to categorize women into groups based on these additional diagnoses. Depression is often secondary to postpartum OCD or panic. If all women with postpartum emotional disorders are lumped together for research purposes, the picture will remain unclear.

Regardless of these problems in the research, interest in postpartum depression remains high, as evidenced by the significant numbers of published studies on the topic (Whiffen, 1992). Most of these researchers agree that postpartum depression may be mild (Hopkins et al., 1989; O'Hara et al., 1990; Pop et al., 1993; York et al., 1992). Affonso et al. (1992) found that only 5% of women met criteria for clinical depression, but a full 50% of the subjects reported clinical levels of three or more relevant depressive symptoms. Anger, fatigue, psychic anxiety, and worry were the most frequent symptoms, and the investigators labeled this as "dysphoric distress." Not only are new mothers plagued by this dysphoria, but poor social and marital adjustment are identified fairly frequently (O'Hara et al., 1990). Attention to the psychological distress, social and/or marital maladjustment is warranted even when mild.

Krause and Redman (1986) suggest that, as for most normal developmental crises, childbearing is a time of risk but is routinely labeled as "wonderful." While they assert that there are incredible stresses associated with this "growth crisis," great anxiety and guilt may arise when the new mother finds that her experience is not fitting with this myth. Kalmuss, Davidson, and Cushman (1992) conducted a test of what they called the "violated expectations hypothesis," comparing women's expectations of parenthood during pregnancy with their actual postbirth experiences. Adjustment to parenthood was significantly more difficult when women's expectations exceeded their experience. Whiffen (1988) looked prospectively at vulnerability to postpartum depression. Prenatal optimistic expectations for the infant predicted depressive symptoms in the postpartum period. Women with unrealistic positive expectations were more likely to exhibit postpartum distress than were women who had accurate expectations about the realities of postpartum life (Atkinson & Rickel, 1984). Our culture and the popular media set up the expectation that having a new baby is "one of the most wonderful times in your life." New families hear this sentiment echoed from numerous sources: television, health professionals, grandparents, and literature from the hospital or baby store. Slade et al. (1993) assessed expectations prenatally, compared these with postnatal reports of experience, and found that expectations of positive emotions greatly exceeded actual experience. The contrast between the cultural expectation that childbirth and early parenting is wonderful and rewarding, and the reality of dysphoric distress and social maladjustment for many women causes intense guilt and feelings of failure (Gruen, 1993). Women who are experiencing negative feelings often ask themselves or professionals, "What is the matter with me for feeling this way?" "Motherhood is supposed to be a happy, fulfilling time," they think, "and if I do not feel that way it must be a flaw in me" (Dix, 1985). Coffman, Levitt, and Brown (1994) tested the effect of confirmation of expectations, finding that when expectations fit with reality, new parents had greater positive affect, relationship satisfaction, and parenting attitudes. Education and normalization about what some 50% of new mothers experience is freeing for these women, decreasing distress (Halonen & Passman, 1985; Whiffen, 1988).

The impact of maternal depression on the mother-child attachment and on the child's development is another reason that postpartum distress should not be ignored or left untreated. The negative effects of the mother's depression on the parent-child relationship have been well-documented (Field et al., 1990; E. M. Zekoski, O'Hara, & Wills, 1987). Having a mother who is experiencing significant emotional distress affects the child's development in many deleterious ways (Downey & Coyne, 1990; Murray, Cooper, & Stein, 1991). The picture is not always as bad as it seems. Philipps and O'Hara (1991) found no direct relationship between postpartum depression and child behavior problems. However, a correlation exists between depression occurring after the postpartum period and child behavior problems, and between postpartum depression and later depression, providing an indirect link between postpartum depression and later child behavior problems. Intervention for mothers with postpartum depression may help to reduce the adverse effects on their children in the long run.

Postpartum distress, if left unrecognized or untreated, may continue, worsen, or recur (Philipps & O'Hara, 1991). In a prospective study of 119 first-time mothers, Kumar and Robson showed that for some women, "Childbearing heralds the start of prolonged emotional difficulties" (1984, p. 44). Some mothers who became depressed for the first time after childbirth continued to experience emotional problems for up to 4 years after the birth. Cooper et al. (1988) had similar continuance rates in their sample. While the prevalence of depression in the first 6 months postpartum is not any greater than in a comparable 6-month period for nonchildbearing women, Cox, Murray, and Chapman (1993) showed onset of depression during the first 5 weeks postpartum to be three times higher. This significant increase in onset during this vulnerable time calls for attention to the problem.

As Whiffen and Gotlib (1993) contend, the average childbearing age coincides with the median age of onset for a first depressive episode, making postpartum depression the first identifiable episode of depression in an adult woman's life. Given that women who suffer from postpartum depression are at increased risk for recurrence (Kumar & Robson, 1984; Philipps & O'Hara, 1991), intervention with these women may not only resolve current difficulties, but prevent the development of subsequent problems.

Increased recognition and attention to postpartum emotional disorders have been fueled by the creation and growth of peer self-help networks. The two principal organizations in the United States are Depression After Delivery and Postpartum Support International (see Table 1 below for addresses and phone numbers). Similar associations exist in nearly every industrialized nation. These grassroots groups have disseminated information through conferences, newsletters, media appearances, and support groups. There continues to be a stigma attached to postpartum emotional problems, with women reluctant or ashamed to admit when their postpartum experience does not fit with the culturally prescribed "positive" model (Gruen, 1993; Knops, 1993). Postpartum Support International and Depression After Delivery work to disarm this stigma, enabling women to feel like valuable human beings and good mothers in spite of negative postpartum emotions.

TABLE 1: RESOURCE LIST
Resources for Self-Help Groups and Professional Education:
Depression After Delivery — National P.O. Box 1282 Morrisville, PA 19067 (215) 295-3994 (800) 944-4PPD
Postpartum Support International 927 N. Kellogg Ave. Santa Barbara, CA 93111 (805) 967-7636
The Marcé Society c/o Michael O'Hara, PhD Department of Psychology University of Iowa Iowa City, IA 52242 (319) 335-2405

CHILDBIRTH: NORMAL BIOLOGICAL
AND PSYCHOSOCIAL CHANGES

Beginning in early pregnancy, the woman experiences a myriad of discomforts related to the hormonal and physical changes in her body. Levels of progesterone and estrogen increase dramatically, rising to 20 to 30 times the normal level by the second trimester (Ford, 1992). Prolactin and adrenal hormone levels are magnified. She experiences extreme physical changes as her uterus, chest, and breasts grow heavy. The amount of blood circulating in her body doubles. These changes are all slow and gradual, over the course of 40 weeks, but result in a feeling that hers is a body other than her own.

At birth, these changes reverse with dramatic speed. Progesterone falls to zero within 1 week. Estrogen declines to 1/200th of pregnancy levels. Prolactin levels increase to aid the production of breast milk and inhibit her body's production of progesterone, estrogen, and other hormones of the endocrine system such as cortisol (Filer, 1992). Even if she chooses not to breast feed her baby, prolactin levels stay high for up to 2 months, delaying the return of progesterone and estrogen to normal levels for some time. The new mother is hungry, fatigued, and perhaps has chills and/or a fever as a reaction to the hard work of labor and birth. She may be in pain from continued contractions, perineal bruises, tears, stitches, or hemorrhoids. Her gastrointestinal tract is sluggish from the effects of the progesterone, making constipation likely. The muscles of the birth canal are soft and enlarged, affecting her control of urination. When her milk "comes in," her breasts get larger, firmer, and increasingly tender, even painful at times. The new mother's changed body often affects her self-image. Many postpartum women voice betrayal by their bodies, which do not function or respond in ways to which the women are accustomed. Although these changes will diminish with time, the new mother needs to feel comfortable with her body in its changed state. Gjerdingen et al. (1993) found that new mothers continue to have physical symptoms well into the first postpartum year, including breast problems, fatigue, hemorrhoids, poor appetite, constipation, increased sweating, acne, numbness and tingling of the hands, hot flashes, and respiratory ailments.

Postpartum physiological adjustment has been likened to post-surgical recovery (Iles, Gath, & Kennerley, 1989; Levy, 1987). With surgery, a patient may have more accurate expectations about the physiological ramifications. Childbirth, on the other hand, is usually viewed as a healthy, normal event. These physical discomforts and dysfunction may be more surprising and unnerving. As one new mother said, echoing many others, "I thought after labor and delivery I was home free; I had no idea of what was ahead of me" (Dunnewold & Sanford, 1994, p. 57). The physical changes occur before the real work of taking care of an infant sets in, adding immense fatigue from lack of sleep to the physical challenges of a postpartum body.

Psychologically, numerous postpartum shifts are required of the family, especially with a first birth. (In this section, mothers will be the focus in wording, but fathers are subject to these same issues.) These emotional changes are as normal as the physical challenges, as the new parents learn to juggle the newborn's needs, continuing relationships with partner and family, and work, household, and social responsibilities (Affonso & Arizmendi, 1986). Becoming a parent signals, individually and culturally, a true step into adulthood, requiring the greatest day-to-day responsibility yet encountered (Greenberg, 1985). Expectations for this maturational process shape us immensely, as new parents often voice: "I really had to grow up now; I had another life depending on me." The developmental process of becoming a mother forces a woman to focus on identity issues. She must decide "Who am I as a mother?" and reconcile this against her former self-image, models she has observed including her own mother, and ideals she may hold for what a mother can or should be. Self-esteem is challenged; her sense of confidence from the work world may generalize easily, or she may suddenly feel that she can do nothing "right" facing this small human being and having no definitive instruction manual. She may have fears about being able to raise the new baby, from worries about accomplishing the day-to-day tasks to providing guidance and structure so the child will grow up healthy and happy (Stern, 1986). She must come to grips with who she wants to be and the strengths which she possesses that transfer to this new role.

Coming to terms with the experience of birth is necessary in the postpartum period (Affonso & Arizmendi, 1986). The first birth is a qualitatively new experience for a woman (Slade et al., 1993). A woman may have information about the birth process and medical interventions, but little appreciation for the reality of either. Many women must process their experiences, finding ways to fit what happened into their schemas about themselves and medical care in general. The new mother may develop expectations for her "performance," feeling she has failed. She may find the experience dehumanizing, feeling like "a piece of meat in a meat market" (Kendall-Tackett & Kantor, 1993, p. 39), fitting a "traumagenic" model. One woman may be deeply affected by physical damage during the birth, another by how she feels different or embarrassed. She may feel betrayed by what she expected versus what actually happened or by her powerlessness and lack of control during the birth (Kendall-Tackett & Kantor, 1993).

The new parents' perception of control over the environment is shaken by parenthood. Prior to the birth, a new parent may feel that he or she really exercises control over his or her world. Beginning with the physical changes of pregnancy (or with the process of achieving pregnancy), it becomes apparent that this control may be an illusion. Before becoming parents, their days were under their control, focused on their needs to eat, sleep, and socialize. Suddenly, someone else's needs take top priority. The baby makes his or her needs well-known and demands immediate response. Balance of the parents' own and the baby's needs becomes paramount. Barraged with cultural messages about putting children first, the new parents often neglect their own needs to the point of physical and/or emotional exhaustion. Babies eat, cry, and sleep on their own schedules, not those of mom, dad, doctor, or grandma. Frantically trying to get the baby to sleep so she can eat even a piece of toast drives this fact home quickly for the new mother. She fears she has lost all control forever, rather than seeing the relative, time-limited nature of parenting an infant.

Lifestyles often must be altered as the new parents face this developmental stage. Without a baby, the parents (individually or as a couple) may have come and gone as they pleased. They may have kept late hours, traveled frequently, slept late, and been unconcerned about the future, financially or otherwise. Now they may feel the pressure of planning before they go out, worrying about the state of the world into which they have brought this child, and/or thinking about college and retirement plans. Values may be reevaluated as the new parents look at the bigger picture of their actions and attitudes with a child in mind (Stern, 1986). These changes come easily for some individuals, and they represent a real sense of loss for others.

Finally, becoming a parent requires changes in the relationships in one's life, whether in the marital/partner relationship, extended family relationships, or friendships. The amount of time which the couple, family, or friends had to devote to each other previously may now be focused on the baby; resulting in feelings of anger and resentment as partners, family members, or friends feel abandoned, neglected, or extraneous. Failed expectations also play a role. The couple may have planned to share parenting responsibilities, only to find that their plan crumbles in the face of reality. In the family-of-origin, the new parent may have hoped to attain a level equal to their parents, or derive via the child, the love and acknowledgment they never received. Siblings may become closer, especially if both are parents and can identify with each other's parenting tasks, providing support. Or having a baby may fire up old rivalry, as the grandparents shift attention to the new baby and away from the adult children. Friendships change, too. Friends with children may welcome the new parents as allies, or shy away as they see competition and challenge for their parenting. Childless friends may resent the efforts and energy that the child takes, feeling it detracts from the relationship. The new parent(s) may have a great need for social support, and be unable to give much back initially.

The normal biological changes in the pregnancy and postpartum period are rivaled by those of adolescence, but are squeezed into a much smaller time frame. Overall, health professionals recognize the crisis dimensions of adolescence, in terms of biological and psychosocial changes, while minimizing the impact of the same degree of changes in new mothers. Culturally, this skewed perspective means that this important time of transition is overlooked by health professionals. Acknowledging the importance of these adjustments for new families, the toll these changes take, and the necessity of support or intervention in this transition to parenthood can help many families cope with this normal, but stressful, time in their lives.

THE BIOLOGICAL BASIS OF POSTPARTUM DISORDERS

The effect of the profound hormonal and endocrinological changes of birth on postpartum emotional disorders has been explored in research. Hopkins, Marcus, and S. B. Campbell (1984) and Filer (1992) both suggest that an indirect, if not direct, connection of these biological changes to postpartum mood makes sense. The considerable endocrinological changes in pregnancy in the hypothalamic-pituitary-adrenal axis may be influential, as in endogenous depression (Smith & Singh, 1992). Research comparing the hormonal changes in women who experience some postpartum mood disturbance and women who do not has been largely equivocal. In these studies, the blues are often studied, based on the assumption that blues predict or precede depression (O'Hara, Schlechte, Lewis, & Wright, 1991).

Handley and associates (Handley et al., 1977, 1980) found disturbances in tryptophan levels and/or their regulation in women who were suffering from postpartum depression. They surmised that this was due to rapid alterations in steroid hormone levels that occur at parturition. Harris et al. (1989) examined 147 mothers at the sixth to eighth week postpartum for levels of cortisol, estradiol, progesterone, and prolactin. They found significant correlations between depression ratings and salivary progesterone and prolactin, especially in breast- versus bottle-feeding mothers. Blood prolactin levels were inadequate in depressed breast-feeding mothers. In a follow-up study, Harris et al. (1994) showed a modest association between scores for maternity blues and changes in salivary progesterone levels. The blues were most likely in women with high prenatal progesterone, low postpartum progesterone, meaning a steep fall in progesterone concentration after delivery. Steinberg (1995) reported a similar finding with pregnant women. Women who developed depression at 36 to 38 weeks gestation had the highest level of a progesterone metabolite, and 80% of these women went on to develop postpartum blues and/or depression.

In a prospective study of the postpartum blues, O'Hara, Schlechte, Lewis, and Wright (1991) followed 182 women from the second trimester of pregnancy through postpartum week 9, assessing levels of progesterone, prolactin, estradiol, free and total estriol, and free and total cortisol. They reported weak support for the hormonal hypothesis that estrogen withdrawal is a cause of postpartum blues, but no support for the role of any of the other hormones they studied. Women with the blues compared to women without the blues had significantly higher free estriol levels at 38 weeks gestation and a significantly greater decrease from mean prepartum levels at day 1 postpartum. O'Hara and colleagues suggested that their measurement of cortisol levels was taken too early to accurately assess the effect of these levels on postpartum mood. Work by Handley et al. (1980) found that high cortisol at 38 weeks gestation was related to depressed mood postpartum. Chrousos (1995) asserts that pregnancy shuts off production of the needed corticotropin-releasing hormone (CRH), the hormone which prompts release of cortisol. In this study of 13 women, CRH secretion by the hypothalamus remained low for as long as 12 weeks after birth. This temporary hormonal deficit could explain low postpartum mood. However, studies by Bonnin

(1992) and Harris et al. (1994) failed to find any significant association between prenatal or postpartum cortisol levels and mood.

Another factor pointing in the direction of a biological link is the finding by O'Hara and colleagues (O'Hara et al., 1990) that one of the best predictors of postpartum blues was a family history of depression or anxiety. This would suggest an inherited biological factor. A previous episode of postpartum depression also increases a woman's risk of developing depression with a subsequent birth (Gitlin & Pasnau, 1989).

Clinicians who work with postpartum women recognize that there are some women who have no psychosocial risk factors for postpartum emotional difficulties, but do suffer greatly with mood changes (Gitlin & Pasnau, 1989). Fernandez (1992) stresses the large numbers of women who have previously been highly functioning individuals. Sichel (1992) and Susman and Katz (1988) point to the clear onset of depression when breast-feeding mothers wean their infants. Joyce, Rogers, and Anderson (1981) detailed onset of mania with weaning. With weaning, the hormonal balance gained during breast feeding is upset. Clinical experience has shown that similar patterns of disorders are evident in some women after pregnancy loss, from miscarriage to molar pregnancy to stillbirth. All these factors support the role of biochemical changes, at least for some women.

As at other times in a person's life (Haggerty et al., 1993; Tallis, 1993), clinical or subclinical hypothyroidism can be responsible for emotional distress in the postpartum period. Following birth, the level of thyroid hormones falls below prepregnancy levels. In some women, the thyroid is slow in returning to its appropriate level of function, and hypothyroidism may result. This is often missed because it is subclinical (Fernandez, 1992), but still causes the woman significant feelings of sluggishness, depression, and exhaustion. Thyroid gland antibodies developed in 38% of one postpartum sample (Harris et al., 1992). Of women with antibodies, 43% reported poor mental health, compared to only 28% of the women without antibodies. Thyroid difficulties need to be ruled out in postpartum women with mood problems.

Postpartum hypopituitarism, or Sheehan's syndrome, is a rare condition that affects a new mother's postpartum mood. The vascular system in late pregnancy is in a sensitive state, and if a patient goes into shock, blood can be obstructed to any bodily organ and cause tissue death. In Sheehan's syndrome, there may be blood loss from ante- or postpartum hemorrhage, or retained or abruptio placenta, which interrupts blood flow to the pituitary and causes a failure in function (J. C. Davis & Abou-Saleh, 1992). When the pituitary fails, the thyroid, adrenals, and ovaries decrease their function. Symptoms include apathy, physical and mental slowdown, cessation of lactation, inability to tan, impaired memory, and loss of libido. Treatment involves administering the hormones which are at low levels in the body. Even though rare, there is evidence that a short period of partial hypopituitarism occurs frequently after childbirth, resulting in a milder set of symptoms (J. C. Davis & Abou-Saleh, 1992).

Postpartum psychosis is likely of biological origin. Evidence of this comes from the work of Nomura and Okano (1992) and Hamilton and Sichel (1992). These physicians have reported effective use of hormones to treat women who have a history of postpartum psychosis. Nomura and Okano reported that postpartum psychosis has been effectively treated with thyroid hormone, or with thyroid hormone combined with antidepressant medication. Hamilton and Sichel (1992) related successful experience with estrogen in preventing the recurrence of postpartum psychosis.

PSYCHOSOCIAL RISK FACTORS FOR POSTPARTUM EMOTIONAL DISORDERS

Childbearing is a time of risk as relationships with self and others are renegotiated (Krause & Redman, 1986). Expectations for this phase of life play a role, as women struggle to meet what may be an unrealistic, idealized standard of a mother who nurtures selflessly, is always in control, loves unconditionally, effortlessly manages a house, children, a full-time job, and meets the demands of her partner (Adcock, 1993). As women come up against these expectations and find they cannot meet them, this reality may compound their feelings of distress, depression, anger, anxiety, and guilt. Research cited previously has shown that these positive expectations are associated with increased depressive symptoms in the postpartum period (Atkinson & Rickel, 1984; Kalmuss et al., 1992; Whiffen, 1988). There are additional factors which increase a woman's chances of having difficulty with this transition.

Having a personal or family history of emotional difficulties increases the risk of developing a postpartum emotional disorder (Gjerdingen & Chaloner, 1994; Whiffen, 1992). Paykel et al. (1980) discovered the woman's psychiatric history to be predictive, independent of other life stressors. J. P. Watson et al. (1984) identified either personal or family history as predictive of postpartum emotional distress. O'Hara and colleagues (O'Hara, Neunaber, & E. M. Zekoski, 1984; O'Hara, Schlechte, Lewis, & Varner, 1991) found the number of previous episodes of depression to be a significant predictor of diagnosis and symptom levels in their childbearing sample. S. B. Campbell et al. (1992) established that a history of affective disorders for a new mother or her first-degree relative predicted the severity of postpartum depression 2 months after birth. Demyttenaere et al. (1995) found that depressive coping style during pregnancy was related to high depression levels at 6 months, but not 6 weeks, after delivery. Having symptoms of anxiety or depression during pregnancy is predictive of postpartum distress as well (Gotlib et al., 1989, 1991; Hobfoll et al., 1995; Pfost, Stevens, & Lum, 1990).

Early childhood experiences play a role in increasing a new mother's risk of developing postpartum difficulties. Frommer and O'Shea (1973) stated that women who had been separated from either parent, through death or divorce, were more vulnerable to depression after the birth of a baby than were those who had no such history. Gotlib et al. (1991) found that women who were depressed postpartum were more likely to perceive as negative the parental care they had received during childhood.

Research addressing the relationship of demographic characteristics to postpartum distress has been mixed. A recent, large-scale study of primiparous women by Gjerdingen and Chaloner (1994) identified young age and low income as significant predictors of postpartum distress. Whiffen (1992) states that age may not be as important as parity (i.e., whether a birth is the woman's first or not), for primiparous women (having their first child) have a greater psychiatric risk (Bebbington et al., 1991). The average age of childbearing women is close to the median age at which individuals experience their first depressive episode (Whiffen, 1992); therefore, studies which identify age as a risk factor may actually be finding that to be true because primiparous women, who are usually younger, are the subjects.

Older research was equivocal regarding postpartum distress and income (Kendall-Tackett & Kantor, 1993; Whiffen, 1992). More recent studies have found that income is a factor, particularly with distress during pregnancy. These studies are somewhat different from previous work, following subjects other than white, middle-class women. Hobfoll and colleagues (1995) identified a postpartum depression rate of 23.4% in their sample of 192 inner-city, impoverished women. This rate is approximately double the rate found in most middle-class samples. E. Watson and Evans (1986) tracked three groups of women, indigenous Britons, and immigrants such as Vietnamese and Bengali natives. While depression occurred in all three groups, the low-income immigrant groups experienced distress that lasted past the first postpartum year. York et al. (1992) followed a mixed race group across pregnancy. Distress, including hostility, was significantly higher among low income, minority women. The importance of making the distinction of onset of depression during pregnancy or after the birth was pointed out by Gotlib et al. (1989). Women whose depression began during pregnancy and continued into the postpartum were younger, less well-educated, and had more children in their households. Finally, in a sample evaluated by S. B. Campbell and Cohn (1991), postpartum distress was related to lower educational level and lesser paternal occupational level. These authors

concluded that their sample size ($N = 1,033$) enabled them to identify small differences, compared to many studies with fewer subjects.

As with depression occurring at other times, postpartum depression appears to be related to stressful life events. Most of the
research by O'Hara and colleagues (O'Hara, Rehm, & S. B.
Campbell, 1982, 1983; O'Hara, 1986; O'Hara, Schlechte, Lewis,
& Varner, 1991; O'Hara, Schlechte, Lewis, & Wright, 1991) has
shown that the greater the number of stressful life events the woman
experiences, the greater her risk for postpartum distress. Both
Bonnin (1992) and Pfost et al. (1990) related stresses of the
pregnancy (hospitalization, weight gain, health problems) to postpartum mood. Gotlib et al. (1991) stated that *perceived* stress,
rather than an actual count of stressful events, was the significant
factor. J. P. Watson et al. (1984) asserted that influential stressors could be acute or chronic, current or past, and related or
unrelated to pregnancy. Whiffen (1988) identified prenatal stress
levels as predictive of postpartum distress. C. P. Cowan and
P. A. Cowan (1987) discovered that the most salient factor is not
the stress level itself, but rather the available support to cope with
that stress level.

It follows that the quality of the woman's social support system is important in postpartum depression. As Kruckman (1992)
reports, postpartum depression does not occur in societies where
instrumental support and aid for the new mother is part of the
cultural tradition. O'Hara et al. (1983) found that depressed
women received less instrumental and emotional support from
members of their social networks than nondepressed controls.
Cutrona (1984) studied support and stress during the transition to
parenthood and found two groups of women were most vulnerable to postpartum depression: women who lacked someone upon
whom to rely for help in any circumstance (reliable alliance), and
women who did not feel themselves part of a social group (social
integration). Affonso and Arizmendi (1986) reiterated this need
to socialize and have a support network for practical aid and advice in their exploratory study. Women who reported difficulties

in resocializing with other adults were more likely to report depressive symptoms. Gjerdingen and Chaloner (1994) found that postpartum depressed women had fewer social supports and fewer recreational activities. Cutrona and Troutman (1986) looked at support and the stressor of infant temperament, and showed that social support protected against the negative effect of difficult infant temperament. Barnett and Parker (1985) studied highly anxious primiparous women, providing social support via either professional social workers or nonprofessional role models who were experienced mothers. This intervention significantly lowered levels of anxiety in this population. Collins et al. (1993) examined the impact of social support on birth outcome and postpartum depression in a sample of low-income pregnant women. Women who reported lower levels of support, particularly from the baby's father, and who had fewer network resources exhibited greater depressed mood during pregnancy and the postpartum. Women with greater levels of support not only experienced less depression, but they had better labor progress and higher Apgar scores for their babies. These researchers discovered that when prenatal life events were low in stress, the amount of support received was unrelated to depression. However, when life events were high in stress, the women with more support were significantly less depressed. Wolman et al. (1993) explored the effects of emotional support during labor on postpartum depression. The women in their study who had a volunteer companion stay with them throughout labor and delivery reported less anxiety and depression than the women without the companion. This was true not just during the birth, but continued for 6 weeks afterwards.

Negative birth events are tied to an increased risk of postpartum emotional distress. Older research has been equivocal, some finding a significant negative association and some a significant positive association. Hannah et al. (1992) found that, in the first postpartum week, low birth weight of the baby, delivery by Caesarean section, a more difficult delivery than expected, and bottle-feeding were all significantly associated with depression scores on the Edinburgh Postnatal Depression Scale (EPDS; Cox,

Holden, & Sagovsky, 1987). At 6 weeks postpartum however, only bottle feeding and Caesarean birth continued to be correlated with EPDS scores. Edwards, Porter, and Stein (1994) studied 300 women, half of whom had delivered by Caesarean section. A significant increase in postpartum depression was noted in the women who had C-sections, though it was a milder illness and tended to begin sooner than depression in women who had vaginal births. S. B. Campbell and Cohn (1991) discovered a connection between even minor obstetric complications and postpartum depression in their sample ($N = 1,033$). Burger et al. (1993) reported a depression rate 2.5 times greater for women with serious medical complications during pregnancy compared to women with no complications. It is not the birth or complications themselves that affect depression in the postpartum period, but rather the impact of those events for the woman (Affonso & Arizmendi, 1986; Arizmendi & Affonso, 1987). Women who are preoccupied by the birth and view it as a stressful event are likely to have more difficulty adjusting in the postpartum period than women who take it in stride.

The quality of a couple's marriage affects the woman's vulnerability to postpartum emotional distress (O'Hara & E. M. Zekoski, 1988). The marriage represents a source of social support. While Whiffen and Gotlib (1993) found that postpartum depressed women had better marital relationships than their sample of nonpostpartum depressed women, most research has demonstrated the opposite to be true. Whiffen (1988) identified low marital adjustment to be predictive of postpartum depression, a finding later confirmed by Gotlib et al. (1991). Path analysis conducted by Demyttenaere et al. (1995) indicated that poor spousal support was a significant predictor of depression at 6 months postpartum. Arizmendi and Affonso (1987) discovered that one of the most intense stressors named by postpartum women was concern about the status of their marital relationship. Being single was identified in three studies as a factor which may increase risk of prenatal or postpartum distress (Feggetter & Gath, 1981; Hobfoll et al., 1995; Pfost et al., 1990).

The effect of employment or length of maternity leave has been investigated in a few studies. Women who listed their occupation as housewife were overrepresented in a group of depressed women (Gotlib et al., 1989). Most other researchers have asserted that there is a negative effect of returning to work, rather than positive. Pop et al. (1993) stated that the period of greatest depression was at 10 weeks postpartum, the end of maternity leave in The Netherlands. At 10 weeks, women who were returning to their jobs had to leave their infants, while women who had chosen not to return to work outside the home had to come to terms with their decision. Gjerdingen and Chaloner (1994) had similar findings: poor mental health in the postpartum year was significantly related to longer work hours and having a maternity leave of less than 24 weeks.

The infant can be another influence on the mother's postpartum emotions. Cutrona and Troutman (1986) looked at the temperament of the infant, with path analysis indicating that the more difficult the infant, the more depressed the mother. In their study, infant difficulty was judged by outside observers. Infant-related stressors (maternal perception of temperament and medical complications) discriminated between depressed and nondepressed mothers in a study by Hopkins, S. B. Campbell, and Marcus (1987). S. B. Campbell et al. (1992) asserted that it is the mother's subjective perception of the baby's temperament which is important, rather than an objective rating. This was the finding in Whiffen's (1988) study as well. Affonso and Arizmendi (1986) found that negative affect while with the baby influenced postpartum depressive symptoms. Having an infant who is ill or otherwise at-risk impacts a new mother's emotional well-being. Bennett and Slade (1991) showed that postpartum emotional distress was predicted by neonatal risk and dissatisfaction with social support from the infant's father. Miller et al. (1993) evaluated crying and fussing data on newborns. They reported that mothers of babies who cried more were more likely to report negative affect. Parker and Barrett (1992) linked infant crying and difficult temperament to Type A behavior in mothers. Mothers who were rated Type A on job involvement had infants who cried more and were rated more difficult. These two studies raise the question of direction of influence: Is the relationship difficult because the mother is depressed/Type A, so her infant cries more? Or when an infant cries more, the mother is more depressed or more invested in her job?

One factor which may mediate with mothers of ill or difficult infants is competence, or self-efficacy, as a parent. Cutrona and Troutman (1986) suggested that one consequence of caring for a difficult infant over time may be an erosion of feelings of competence as a parent. Women who had high levels of social support appeared to be buffered from the effect of caring for a demanding infant, primarily through the mediation of self-efficacy. Clinical experience with mothers of at-risk infants has demonstrated this, as well. Mothers who must take a nursing, rather than a parenting, role with an ill infant often question their abilities as caretakers, because the tasks they must perform are not consistent with their expectations of what parenting involves.

Attributional style, perfectionism, and need for control appear to be influential in the mother's vulnerability to postpartum emotional distress (Fernandez, 1992). Negative attributional/coping style during pregnancy was related to mood at 2 to 6 months in three studies (Cutrona, 1984; Demyttenaere et al., 1995; O'Hara et al., 1982). Pfost and colleagues (1990) showed that antepartum depressive symptoms were predictive, using multiple regression analysis, of postpartum depression. Donovan and colleagues (Donovan & Leavitt, 1989; Donovan, Leavitt, & Walsh, 1990) examined two groups of mothers, assessing illusory control. Women with high illusory control were more likely to feel depressed, incompetent as parents, and to experience guilt over not being "perfect mothers." While research has minimized the predictive value of characteristics such as these compared to other factors such as family or personal history of depression or social support, in clinical experience these attributes are extremely important. Many couples work to control their lives and do everything in the "right" order, finishing education, establishing a career, and so forth. The reality of infant care and the lack of control involved can be extremely disruptive. Babies decide to be born, sleep, eat, cry, and dirty their diapers on their own schedules, and for many people this is the first encounter with a lack of control in their lives. This lack of control thus becomes extremely upsetting and crucial to the parents.

The contribution of any of these risk factors likely varies from individual to individual, and the cause of postpartum distress is best seen as multifactorial. It seems probable that the biological changes of pregnancy and birth may kindle some biochemical vulnerability in many women (Parry, 1992). Life stresses, social support, and individual expectations and characteristics add to the equation. The lack of societal support and structure for new families should not be neglected (LoCicero, Weiss, & Issokson, 1995). The normal adjustment becomes too much for her resources, overwhelming the new mother and resulting in significant emotional distress.

WHO IS MOST VULNERABLE?
CLINICAL EXPERIENCES

In clinical practice, the new mother who is most likely to experience some postpartum distress has numerous risk factors. The following examples illustrate the multitude of factors influencing postpartum distress for many women.

Vignette #1

Judy,* age 32, developed some depression during pregnancy, after moving from the large metropolitan area where she had lived since college to another large metropolitan area halfway across the country. Married for 2 years, Judy was relocating because of her husband's career, which meant putting her own career on hold. The physical stresses of relocating on top of the pains of late pregnancy had exhausted

---

* Name and all identifying characteristics of persons in all case examples have been disguised thoroughly to protect privacy.

her. Knowing no one in the new city, she slept through most of the end of pregnancy, having contact only with her husband. She lacked a social support system, and had a husband heavily invested in his career. He was very traditional, and saw childcare as Judy's job, especially since she was not currently employed outside the home.

Judy had previously experienced depression and had received counseling after her parents had divorced 6 years earlier. Because her family lived 1,000 miles away, they were unavailable to help with the new baby. Judy had little experience with infants, and was a very verbal person. Home with the baby all day long, she quickly became frustrated with the realities of infant care. She had no one to talk to. The baby did not seem to communicate in a way she could decipher; and there was no break in sight. Judy was used to controlling her life and doing things on her own timetable, which seemed completely lost in this new role. She felt she had sacrificed her "career" self for an unrewarding "life of drudgery." She became increasingly depressed, failed to get dressed, had difficulty sleeping, and continued to "eat for two." She also had extreme angry outbursts: throwing things and yelling at her husband for taking her away from her home and not providing any breaks from this baby. Because she had sought help with her depression before, Judy was aware of her difficulties, and took steps to get the help she needed.

Vignette #2

Carla was a 34-year-old, married, mother of three. She had experienced some slight depression with her first child, in which she found herself frequently tearful over the trials and tribulations of life with a new baby. Through this first postpartum period she had lived in a fog, until slowly the anxiety and overwhelming feelings lifted on their own. With the birth of the third baby, Carla was caring for the two older children, now 7 and 4 years old, full time. Carla had a few friends, but was reluctant to ask for help. Her mother had a history of emotional problems and was always burdening her friends with her feelings. Because of this, Carla was adamant about not admitting that she had negative feelings to anyone.

The first 3 days home with the new baby, the baby was quite fussy and cried for long periods at night. By the fourth day, Carla's husband returned to work, leaving Carla to care for the children on her own. She was breast feeding, caring for the older children and shuttling them to their activities, and "hurrying all day long." Unwinding after such hectic days was hard, and she was having trouble sleeping. When the baby was 1 week old, Carla's husband had to go out of town overnight on business. The night he was gone, Carla could not sleep at all. Her anxiety about not being able to sleep skyrocketed, making sleep even less likely. She worried day and night. By day 10 of the baby's life, Carla's anxiety had risen to a level she could not control. She cried and worried all night to her husband. She repeatedly voiced the fear that she was "going nuts like my mother" and would never be normal again.

DIAGNOSIS AND TREATMENT

OVERVIEW OF POSTPARTUM EMOTIONAL DISORDERS

Emotional reactions following the birth of a baby are often referred to as "postpartum depression (PPD)," lumping together anything from constant tearfulness on the part of a new mom to the rarer phenomenon of new mothers who have homicidal thoughts about their babies. The more attention paid to postpartum emotions, the more evidence emerges that PPD is not a single, distinct entity. Rather, a full spectrum of emotional symptoms is possible for related but varied postpartum emotional syndromes. Knowing the distinctions and diagnosing properly is extremely reassuring to the woman and her family, and is necessary for appropriate treatment. As Wohlreich (1994) asserts, recognizing postpartum illness is the most important factor in its management.

Normal Postpartum Adjustment and the Blues. The continuum of emotions after the birth of a baby is illustrated in Table 2 (next page). For the majority of new mothers, the biological and

TABLE 2: SPECTRUM OF POSTPARTUM EMOTIONAL DISORDERS*

BABY BLUES	NORMAL ADJUSTMENT	POSTPARTUM EMOTIONAL DISORDERS	POSTPARTUM PSYCHOSIS
◆ Crying	◆ Crying/Tearfulness	◆ Postpartum depression: • Worsening of "normal" symptoms	◆ Any symptoms at left, plus. . .
◆ Irritability	◆ Irritability	◆ Postpartum panic: • panic attacks, new onset • extreme anxiety • physical symptoms: difficulty breathing, dizziness, shaking, and so on	◆ Confusion
◆ Anger	◆ Anger		◆ Hallucinations
◆ Insomnia	◆ Sleep disturbance		◆ Delusions
◆ Exhaustion	◆ Fatigue	◆ Postpartum mania: • feeling "speeded up" • decreased need to sleep • distractibility, pressured speech • irritability, excitability	
◆ Tension	◆ Dysphoria		
◆ Anxiety	◆ Appetite changes	◆ Postpartum stress: • panic attacks related to past trauma	
◆ Restlessness	◆ Loss of interest	◆ Postpartum obsessive-compulsive: • repetitive, intrusive thoughts • thoughts "come out of the blue" • thoughts are repulsive/shocking • avoidance likely, but not ritual	
	◆ Anxiety		
	◆ Emotional lability		
	◆ Feelings of doubt (parenting, etc.)		
	◆ Postpartum exhaustion: • denial of depression or anxiety • feeling overwhelmed • unable to sleep/rest • head or stomachaches		

*Adapted with permission from *Postpartum Survival Guide* by Ann Dunnewold and Diane Sanford. Copyright © 1994 New Harbinger Publications, Inc.

psychosocial changes do not interfere with day-to-day functioning, and are part of the normal adjustment to having a child. Approximately 80% of all women go through the *baby blues,* with symptoms listed in the left-hand column of the chart. The blues are a mild change in mood occurring 24 to 48 hours postpartum, due to the dramatic hormonal changes of labor and childbirth. The blues are self-limiting, resolving on their own as these physical stresses and hormonal changes even out. The blues are so common as to be considered normal, and require only education and support. Women with the blues report crying easily, reacting with irritation over trivialities they would normally ignore, suffering fatigue, having difficulty sleeping, being more emotional than usual, or feeling slight anxiety or agitation. For most women, the baby blues do not last beyond 2 weeks, although some women may have mild symptoms for up to 6 weeks following delivery. *Normal postpartum adjustment* is the extension of the blues symptoms through the first 2 months postpartum. Normal adjustment is a misleading term to the general public, because this degree of negative feeling seems abnormal. Societal expectations do not prepare women for the crying, anger, fatigue, and related feelings which are listed next on the continuum.

Honey Watts, Director of the Calgary Postpartum Support Society (personal communication, June 1993) has suggested that postpartum exhaustion is a distinct category on this adjustment portion of the continuum. In postpartum exhaustion, women feel fairly well psychologically: no depression or anxiety is reported. A woman with postpartum exhaustion feels overwhelmed and "bone-tired," simply unable to function. She may not be sleeping well, during the day or night. Instead of resting, she is busy meeting the needs of her baby, the household, and other family members. She may have physical symptoms, that is, headaches or stomachaches, and may consult medical specialists trying to find a concrete physical malady. Many of the symptoms disappear when the baby begins to follow a regular sleep schedule; the mother then recovers from sleep deprivation. It can take several weeks before the new mother feels like herself again.

Case Example:
Normal Adjustment

Joy was 26 years old, married for 3 years, and content with her job as an accounting clerk when she discovered she was pregnant. The pregnancy and birth went well, and Joy was home from the hospital 36 hours after birth with a healthy, though vocal, baby boy. Joy and her husband, Tim, were both taken aback by how much this baby cried. It seemed like he could wail for 3 hours at a time, and he particularly preferred the hours from 11:00 p.m. to 2:00 a.m.. They spelled each other on this nightly duty, walking the baby as he fussed. Every time they set him down, he would begin to cry again. Joy reported thinking "I have made a terrible mistake."

Joy often became overwhelmed, had a good cry, and went on. When the baby finally slept, she would lie awake worrying about why the baby cried so much. Several times she became panicky, thinking "I will never have a life again." Through the first 3 weeks of the baby's life, she became increasingly tired and irritable. Several times Tim came home from work to find Joy and the baby asleep on the couch together, still in the nightclothes from that morning. He could not understand why she snapped at him so easily, as if he was to blame for all of this.

One day while walking around the neighborhood, Joy saw another mother with a stroller. This neighbor had a 6-month-old baby, as well as a 3 year old. As they talked, Joy began to see that this time in her life was actually very short. Joy had never had such negative feelings before, and meeting this new friend allowed her to see that her positive view of the world need not be lost. As the baby approached 6 weeks of age, his crying began to lessen. Joy began to get more sleep, and discovered that she did not cry so much when she got 6 hours of sleep in a row. It had been a pretty horrible start to being a parent, but by the time the baby was 8 weeks old Joy felt like the good days outweighed the days of crying and anger.

As women and their partners move through the adjustment of the postpartum period, they must come to terms with the self-image, lifestyle, and relationship changes required of this life transition. How she and her partner weather this stage depends on the number of stumbling blocks which occur: marital and other social supports, life stressors, maladaptive expectations for the realities of parenting and their abilities, and guilt over failing to conform to these expectations. These stresses and feelings of fault or failure complicate the normal feelings of the postpartum, making them much more daunting. If her ability to complete daily tasks is affected, or normal symptoms worsen over a 2- to 5-week period, a postpartum disorder may be developing.

In normal adjustment, the good feelings outweigh the negative. When the negative feelings become more powerful and prevalent than the positive feelings, the balance has switched. If a woman is having difficulty with her daily functioning, or the negative feelings appear to be the salient feature in her life — even if she is managing to care for herself and her child — she has moved on the continuum into the range of postpartum disorders.

Postpartum Affective Disorders. Repeated research has shown that postpartum depression strikes from 10% to 20% of new mothers. Figures are not available on postpartum mania; this has not been clearly delineated in the literature to date. Postpartum mania may signal the start of a postpartum psychosis, described later. Many cases of mania may be included in research on psychosis, due to overlap between syndromes. There are women who develop postpartum mania who do not become floridly psychotic. Postpartum psychosis may be an affective psychosis. The onset of postpartum psychosis is often insidious; the new mother may not initially notice impairment in her thinking. Confusion in the postpartum period is not uncommon, given the demands put on the new mother and the sleep deprivation she may face. In very rare instances, postpartum depression can develop into a psychosis, and may put a woman at risk for suicide and/or infanticide.

Postpartum Depression. The onset of postpartum depression is usually slow and gradual, and has an on-again, off-again nature. Postpartum depression begins most often in the first 2 months of the baby's life. Symptoms fluctuate and are heterogeneous (Appleby et al., 1994). The new mother may have extreme changes in appetite and sleep patterns. Difficulty returning to sleep after feeding the baby at night is particularly diagnostic. Tearfulness and crying spells, a short attention span and problems concentrating, and spells of dysphoric mood are common. A lack of energy and loss of interest in enjoyed activities are also characteristic, as are increasing irritability and sensitivity. Even when mild, these feelings are terribly disruptive to the new mother.

Women with postpartum depression admit to feeling helpless and hopeless about their situation. They fear that they do not have it in them to be good mothers, or to ever care for their infants "in the right way." Many new mothers fear that they have lost their familiar "old self" completely. They feel like a burden to their spouse, family, and friends. Faced with nagging self-doubts, many women who previously viewed themselves as competent and successful begin to see themselves as failing and incompetent. Very often this is accompanied by a tremendous sense of guilt about not living up to personal or societal expectations for a good mother. Women say "The baby deserves a better mother than I can ever be." Guilt compounds the worries about the effects of her mood on the baby. Suicidal feelings, or thoughts about harming the baby, can haunt her. *DSM-IV* (American Psychiatric Association, 1994) diagnosis for postpartum depression takes two forms. The milder presentation is most accurately diagnosed as an adjustment disorder, usually with mixed anxious and depressed mood (309.28). *DSM-IV* allows for delineation of major depressive disorder (296.2 or 296.3) with the specifier "with postpartum onset."

Case Example:
Postpartum Depression

Kim was 23 years old, married, and employed part-time as a teacher's aide when she had her first child, a girl. For the first 2 weeks, she took off work and concentrated on caring for the baby. Mari, the baby, slept and nursed well. Kim had a touch of the blues, crying for an hour several times. She had been around children a great deal, and felt quite confident about her ability to be a parent. At the end of 2 weeks, Kim was bored. They needed her at work. Since she worked in a private school, the director let her bring the baby along, keeping her in the teacher's lounge or in the baby front-pack while she was in the classroom. She began to stay at work longer than she needed to and to take on extra projects, because she felt that having the baby with her decreased the amount of work she could accomplish in her regular hours. Kim had always been a perfectionist, and felt she had to prove herself. After work, she cooked dinner, bathed the baby, prepared the next day's projects, and collapsed exhausted by the time her husband arrived home at 8:00 p.m. Kim became increasingly tired and irritable. Two teachers at the school took her aside, telling her she need not work so hard to prove herself. But Kim had high expectations for herself. She was sleeping less and less, and feeling more and more angry. Her husband had only changed about three diapers in this child's life. She had no one to whom she could confide her feelings; she wanted to appear strong to everyone she knew. This lifestyle was taking its toll. She seemed to catch every sniffle and cough that the kids brought to school. At her director's insistence, Kim made an appointment to see a psychologist. It was so foreign to focus on herself that she cried through the first session. She completed 10 counseling sessions and learned it was necessary and permissible to take care of herself first, and ask for help from others.

Postpartum Mania. Postpartum mania appears in the same time frame as the blues, the days immediately postbirth. Women frequently describe themselves as feeling "speeded up"; they have trouble relaxing or slowing down, and exhibit a decreased need for sleep. The new mother may sleep for only 2 or 3 hours a day, without fatigue. Pressured speech, distractibility, and mood swings are common. The manic new mother may appear at first to be productive; she might make lots of lists of things to do, or clean house excessively, or begin any number of difficult projects. These activities are unproductive, as she jumps from one task to another, leaving a wake of chaos behind her. Unlike mania unrelated to childbirth, postpartum mania is not usually characterized by an elated or euphoric mood, but rather irritability and excitability. Initially, impairment in her thinking may be unnoticeable. Faulty reasoning, poor judgment, and distorted perceptions may be minimal, but can quickly progress to an impaired level. Women having symptoms of mania need immediate professional treatment. *DSM-IV* diagnosis identifies the appropriate bipolar disorder; in most cases this is bipolar I disorder, single manic episode (296.0x). As in depressive episodes, "with postpartum onset" is specified to delineate the relationship to the birth.

Case Example: Postpartum Mania

Laura was a 26-year-old married woman who gave birth to a baby girl. Always labeled by her family as "anxious" and "high-strung," she had come to view herself this way. She had no history of treatment, though there was a family history of bipolar disorder. The baby was an "aggressive nurser," initially breast feeding every 1 to 2 hours. Laura did not mind this; it made her feel close to the baby. She was extremely protective, only she could care for the baby. In the first week, Laura felt many self-doubts as her anxiety rose. She began to lose sleep because of the baby's high demands and her worries about handling these new responsibilities. When the baby was 10 days old, she had not slept more than an hour in 3 days. Increasingly irritable with her family, she refused to eat. She denied any difficulties, saying "Just leave me alone and let me take care of my baby." If she was not feeding the baby, she paced the house with her bundled in her arms, leaving the room as soon as any family member tried to talk to her. Laura's family recognized the manic pattern, and immediate psychiatric consultation was arranged. She was quickly stabilized on medication, and able to resume her parental duties with the support of her family and a therapist.

Postpartum Anxiety Disorders. Postpartum anxiety disorders consist of heightened feelings of anxiety and/or panic. These feelings are recurrent and can be vague and nonspecific, focused on life and the world in general or situation-specific. Fears and anxiety-provoking thoughts about the baby are characteristic. Postpartum anxiety disorders include postpartum panic, postpartum obsessive-compulsive disorder, and postpartum stress reaction. Prevalence rates are not available. Clinicians have only recently identified these patterns, and the estimate of 10% to 20% for postpartum depression likely includes anxiety disorders. Anxiety symptoms usually manifest themselves in the first 2 to 3 weeks after the birth of a baby, but may not reach a distressing level until weeks later. If not identified and treated promptly, a woman may become depressed in reaction to her anxious feelings. The typical new mother expects to feel confident and happy after her baby is born, and may wonder if there is something gravely wrong with her for having such scary worries. Self-doubt and guilt over not being able to control the worry can only worsen the common blue feelings of the postpartum period. This secondary depression results in many women in this category being evaluated as depressed for research purposes. Clinically, over 50% of women identify the anxiety as preceding the depression.

Postpartum Panic Disorder. Postpartum panic disorder was first described in the literature by Metz et al. (1988) in three case studies. Sholomskas et al. (1993) investigated whether panic occurring for the first time in the postpartum period was a coincidental event. Of their sample ($N = 64$), seven women (10.9%) met criteria for postpartum onset of panic. This was significantly greater than the expected age-corrected percentage of 0.92%. Onset of panic after the first birth thus was not coincidental. Women with previous panic are at risk of recurrence postpartum.

Women with postpartum panic disorder frequently remark that their panic attacks and anxious feelings "come out of the blue." A panic attack is an episode of extreme anxiety in which a person experiences physical symptoms such as shortness of breath, chest pain or discomfort, choking or smothering sensations, dizziness, tingling in hands or feet, trembling and shaking, sweating, faintness, and hot and cold flashes. During a panic attack, the woman may fear she is dying, going crazy, or losing control. A general sense of restlessness, agitation, or irritability may be present. Symptoms can be continuous or intermittent. The new mother may have difficulty identifying a particular event or situation as the trigger. Lack of a provoking incident increases her helpless, overwhelmed feelings. Many of these women initially visit a hospital emergency room, convinced they are physically ill or having a heart attack. Postpartum women frequently report being wakened from sleep by these symptoms. The new mother may have recurrent fears and thoughts about harm coming to her child(ren), other loved ones, or herself. These obsessive fears can make problems with depression or anxiety even worse. *DSM-IV* diagnosis is usually panic disorder without agoraphobia (300.01). *DSM-IV* does not delineate use of the specifier "with postpartum onset," but that phrase provides clarity if added.

Case Example:
Postpartum Panic Disorder

Linda was 19 years old when she had her first child. She had married her high school sweetheart, anxious to have a family right away. When the baby was 3 days old, Linda became panicky. Initially a shaky feeling inside, it built into a full-fledged panic attack by the time the baby was 3 weeks old. Although she did not have a personal history of anxiety, she did have a family history of it. Linda was fairly unsophisticated at this young age, and merely suffered through these symptoms. She had her second child 8 years later. Pregnancy gave her relief from the panic; but symptoms returned full-force after the birth. It was at this point that Linda sought professional help, finding a therapist through a support group. She was adamant that she be able to continue to breast feed her baby, and so refused to take medication. Through cognitive-behavioral therapy, Linda learned to control and defuse her symptoms.

Postpartum Obsessive-Compulsive Disorder. Postpartum obsessive-compulsive disorder (OCD) has been described in the literature by Neziroglu, Anemone, and Yaryura-Tobias (1992) and Sichel et al. (1993). These researchers have concluded that pregnancy and/or the puerperium may be significant periods of risk for developing new-onset obsessive-compulsive disorder. Sichel (1990) estimated that 3% to 5% of new mothers may develop obsessive symptoms. Recurrence of obsessive symptoms in patients with a previous history is common.

In postpartum OCD, the primary symptom is the occurrence of repetitive and persistent thoughts, ideas, or images. These arise spontaneously, without intentional thought, in the first postpartum weeks. Women report "The thought just popped into my head." Most commonly, these spontaneous and disturbing ideas have to do with harming her baby. Prevalent fantasies include hurting the baby with knives, putting the baby in the microwave oven, suffocating the baby, throwing him or her down stairs, or drowning the child. Women who are survivors of childhood sexual abuse may have thoughts or fantasies of molesting their children in similar ways. Other loved ones, such as an older child, a partner, or a parent, may be the less frequent object of these worries. The possible harm imagined can include accidental events, such as automobile crashes, or illnesses such as cancer. The *DSM-IV* diagnosis obsessive-compulsive disorder (300.3) is most appropriate. As with panic, the specifier "with postpartum onset" may be explanatory.

A less frequent symptom of postpartum OCD is the performance of ritualistic behaviors or compulsions to reduce the anxiety. Women may hide the knives or avoid the kitchen in an effort to ward off thoughts of harming the baby with knives. She may refuse to bathe the baby out of fear of thoughts about death by drowning. Obsessions alone are not more difficult to treat than compulsions (Arts et al., 1993).

Thoughts like these are actually common in new mothers, as they become acutely aware of how vulnerable babies are. Salkovskis and P. Campbell (1994) contend that negative intrusive thoughts occur in more than 80% of the general population. Intrusive thoughts may be this common in new mothers as well, but only a small proportion are disturbed by what such thoughts could mean about their personal integrity and get stuck on the thoughts (Foa, 1992). The new mother may run these disturbing ideas over and over in her head, trying to control and make sense of them, aiming to protect her child in this dangerous world.

Obsessive thoughts cause the woman a great deal of distress and self-loathing, as she asks herself, "What is the matter with me for thinking this way?" Clinical experience suggests that these destructive images may be the result of feelings the new mother is reluctant to acknowledge. Negative feelings that don't fit with a woman's expectations for parenthood may come out indirectly in this manner. If the new mother expects parenthood always to be fun and rewarding, rather than tiring, draining, and frustrating at times, she may become disillusioned with the experience of having a new baby. Anger at her situation, spouse, or other family members may result. She may be so invested in control, perfectionism, and having everything turn out *right* that she cannot acknowledge or accept her anger.

Professional treatment, possibly including medication, is needed if the new mother is not able to dismiss these intrusive ideas. Women with postpartum OCD are *always* clear that these thoughts are wrong, and offensive, and should not be carried out (Sichel et al., 1993). The differences between postpartum OCD and postpartum psychosis are (a) this ability to know that the thoughts are wrong and should not be acted on, and (b) the reaction of disgust that the woman has to her thoughts. Women with postpartum OCD have not been known to carry out their disturbing thoughts, while women with postpartum psychosis are not repulsed by their thoughts and may actually act on them. It is important that health professionals understand this critical distinction, for misdiagnosis can be harmful. If postpartum OCD is confused with postpartum psychosis, the woman may be incorrectly judged to be a danger to her child. Infants have been removed from their mothers by child protective services after this misdiagnosis, causing extreme stress for the mother, the family, and negatively impacting the parent-child attachment. Extreme caution is advised in evaluating mothers with thoughts about hurting their infants, in order to avoid this tragic mistake.

Case Example:
Postpartum Obsessive-Compulsive Disorder

Susan was 37 years old when she had her first child. She had been treated for an obsessive disorder when she was 21 years old. The interval in between was problem-free, and she was unnerved to find herself harboring obsessive thoughts about her 6-week-old baby. She described these thoughts as simply arising out of her frustration one night as the baby cried. The thoughts were about drowning the baby as Susan bathed her, or stabbing the baby with knives as she sat on the kitchen counter in her infant seat. Susan experienced these thoughts as ego dystonic; she was surely a terrible person for having such ideas. She berated herself: She must be a monster, a horrible mother, a sick person. She was intensely concerned that, even though she knew she should not act on these thoughts, when she was tired or stressed she would "slip," and somehow act out her thoughts. She talked to her obstetrician, who recommended a therapist well-respected in the community. Susan saw him one time; in which he questioned her intently about her past, especially any history of violent behavior. Susan left the session feeling even worse; he seemed to be confirming her fears that there was something terribly wrong with her. She struggled through several more weeks, talking about the thoughts with her husband and mother, who tried in vain to reassure her. At that point she saw a television program about postpartum women who have killed their infants. The program upset her terribly, but also gave her the number for Depression After Delivery (DAD), a national support network. Susan called this number and received information about local professional and peer support resources. Susan felt imminently better when she talked to one woman who had survived postpartum OCD. She scheduled an appointment with the professional on the DAD list, and felt reassured about the lack of risk to her infant. After connecting with these resources and receiving this support, Susan felt much better and began to be able to dismiss the thoughts as just thoughts as she had learned to do in the earlier OCD episode.

Postpartum Stress Disorder. Unlike postpartum panic disorder which has no identifiable trigger, women who suffer from postpartum stress disorder can point to a specific event. While the woman may not be immediately aware of the trigger, careful evaluation of the events related to her panic leads to the provoking factors. This may be a recent trauma such as potentially life-threatening complications during labor and delivery; or a trauma from the woman's past. Past traumas include accidents, violent assaults, or even a previous birth, the recollection of which sets off panic in the subsequent pregnancy. A new mother exposed to a situation that reminds her of this trauma is vulnerable to panic attacks. Women having an attack fear that they will die if subjected to the traumatic event a second time. Avoidance may occur. For example, women who fear choking may stop eating solid foods in order to avoid reexperiencing the earlier trauma. The attacks and the avoidance behaviors may be variable over time.

Most postpartum women do not have flashbacks or nightmares when presented with reminders of the trauma, although both can occur. Similarly, the numbing or emotional detachment is usually lacking. This is not always so, as Moleman et al. (1992) describe for partus stress reaction. They relate three cases in which women with histories of infertility and complicated pregnancies experienced panic and dissociative reactions during labor and delivery. Postpartum women may fit the *DSM-IV* categories of posttraumatic stress disorder (309.81) or acute stress disorder (308.3).

Case Example:
Postpartum Posttraumatic Stress Disorder

Rita was a 33-year-old, married, mother of one. She had no prior psychiatric history. The first birth was a dreadful experience. Labor had been 43 hours long. Forceps had been attempted, with vaginal tearing from the forceps, followed by an emergency Cesarean section when the baby's heart rate suddenly dropped. Rita was extremely upset at the time, and postponed a repeat pregnancy for 5 years because of strong feelings about the birth. With the second pregnancy, she had a more understanding physician, who urged her to take a refresher childbirth preparation class. When walking into the hospital for the first class, Rita began to perspire. Thinking it was just due to late pregnancy and the summer heat, she and her husband sat down in the classroom. The instructor began by asking participants to tell their previous birth stories. As Rita listened to the other couples talk, she began to feel dizzy and sick to her stomach. Her hands began to shake. Her palms were sweating. She felt faint, unable to breathe. She closed her eyes and leaned her head on her husband's shoulder. When it was her turn to describe her previous birth, Rita got up and ran from the room, gasping for breath.

The next day she called her physician, who wanted to see her right away to rule out gestational diabetes. As soon as Rita entered the hospital building, where her doctor's office was located, the symptoms began again. The doctor determined that she was suffering panic attacks brought on by the fear of delivery. The doctor arranged for Rita to see a psychologist who helped her deal with her fears through relaxation and imagery, preparing for the birth. Rita and her husband hired a professional labor coach to help reinforce these skills during the labor and birth. Rita came through the birth with a minimum of emotional discomfort, and with the skills she had learned felt in control throughout the birth.

Postpartum Psychosis. Postpartum psychosis is the extreme on the continuum of postpartum emotional disorders, and the rarest of all. Throughout history, rates of postpartum psychosis have been 1 to 2 per 1,000 births. The onset of postpartum psychosis is usually early, within the first 24 to 72 hours after the baby's birth. But it can occur at later times, particularly in conjunction with such physical stresses as weaning or severe sleep deprivation. Rohde and Marneros (1993) set the following criteria: (a) onset of illness within 6 weeks after birth, (b) no previous mental illness, and (c) no psychiatric symptoms during pregnancy. In this study of 86 women, average age was 26.3 years. More than 75% of the mothers were primiparous. In 55.8% of the mothers, first symptoms appeared in the first week postpartum, and in 22.1% first symptoms occurred in the second week postpartum. Paranoid symptoms were present in more than 50% of this group, restlessness in 57%, and catatonic excitement in 44.2%. Anxiety, sleep disturbance, and dysphoria were also frequent symptoms.

A new mother suffering from postpartum psychosis has abnormal thought processes, beyond the mere forgetfulness or spaciness that is common postpartum. She loses touch with reality. Changes in mood may be evident. Symptoms of postpartum psychosis range from moderate to severe, and can progress quite rapidly. Milder symptoms of extreme distractibility and racing thoughts, as in postpartum mania, may herald the onset of the psychosis. Significant confusion, poor judgment, and delusions or hallucinations may exist, which often have a religious quality. For example, a woman may believe that her baby is Jesus, or hear voices telling her that the baby is the Devil. The severity and bizarre nature of these thoughts clearly distinguishes them from the obsessions that make up postpartum OCD. The latter are related to more commonplace, day-to-day activities. And, as stated previously, women with postpartum OCD have not been known to act on their violent thoughts, whereas psychotic women have done so. A woman suffering from psychosis is unclear about the reality of her thoughts, while a woman with OCD is able to clearly tell that her thoughts are wrong, repulsive, and not to be acted upon.

Postpartum psychosis can be life-threatening to both mother and baby; thus immediate and aggressive medical attention is critical. Knops (1993) notes that a 5% rate of suicide and a 4% rate of infanticide have been reported with the disorder. Women with a personal or family history of bipolar illness have a significantly greater risk for developing postpartum psychosis. Monitoring by a mental health professional during pregnancy and following the birth are essential.

Case Example:
Postpartum Psychosis

Amy was a 30-year-old first-time mom. Within 3 days of the birth, she began to feel "strange," crying 1 minute, laughing uncontrollably the next. She began to feel that her husband and her mother were plotting to take the baby away from her. When the baby was 6 days old, she began to hallucinate. Dark forms seemed to swirl around her in the room; she felt like they were demons after the baby. She huddled in her bed, cuddling the baby close. When she refused to get up over the next 24 hours, her family became deeply concerned. She was taken to the emergency room, where she was admitted to the psychiatric unit. She was stabilized quite quickly on antipsychotic medication, and was home in 4 days. With continued support and counseling, Amy was almost completely recovered by the time the baby was 3 months old.

Each disorder is described here as if it existed in some distinct place along the spectrum of disorders. In clinical practice, there is considerable overlap between categories. New mothers may have symptoms from more than one category, or may exhibit varied patterns along the spectrum at different times. Symptoms can begin during pregnancy also, and especially deserve attention then. As noted earlier, similar patterns can be evident after pregnancy loss.

CLINICAL ASSESSMENT

The question of "Why do I not hear about postpartum distress (PPD) in my own work?" is frequently asked by health professionals. The answer may lie in several realms. First of all, a significant stigma still exists about feeling negatively during pregnancy or the postpartum. Women continue to believe, especially with first pregnancies, that the whole experience will be emotionally positive. Thinking they should feel great, excited, and only minimally apprehensive, women routinely question their own mental health and self-worth when their personal experience does not fit this cultural norm. Women repeatedly voice: "I thought there was something the matter with me for feeling this way." These doubts seriously hinder their willingness to reveal negative experiences. Another reason health professionals hear little about postpartum distress is that they are not trained to inquire routinely. They fall prey to the myths about pregnancy and the postpartum period being exclusively positive, and do not ask about postpartum distress. The symptoms of postpartum distress may often be overlooked because they are confused with normal postpartum symptoms involved in caring for a newborn such as weight loss, fatigue, and sleep disturbance (Knops, 1993). Finally, research cited earlier shows that assessments at different times yield various results. It may be that our current health care system, with little contact by the obstetrician from birth to the 6-week checkup, and then contacts with the pediatrician focused on the child, misses the greatest periods of vulnerability.

Assessment Instruments. The Edinburgh Postnatal Depression Scale (EPDS) was developed by Cox, Holden, and Sagovsky (1987). The EPDS has been widely used throughout Great Britain, clinically and in research. The EPDS is a quick screening device, taking only minutes to score. It has been shown in research to have a superior sensitivity and specificity with postpartum women compared to the Beck Depression Inventory (Holden, 1991). One disadvantage is that women have little room to elaborate upon their symptoms, and so it requires follow-up with an in-depth interview. Stein and Van den Akker (1992) have designed the Bromley Postnatal Depression Scale, a screening instrument with the advantage of providing longitudinal information. The woman responds to questions about the current postpartum period, as with the EPDS, and about previous postpartum experiences. These authors report adequate reliability and validity, but caution against relying on this scale as sole criterion. As with the EPDS, follow-up with a clinical interview is needed.

Affonso et al. (1990) refined the Schedule for Affective Disorders and Schizophrenia (SADS; Endicott & Spitzer, 1978) to account for the influence of pregnancy and postpartum physical symptoms. The revised version, which they labeled as SADS-PPG (SADS-Pregnancy and Postpartum Guidelines), corrects some of the problems of over- and underdiagnosis possible when using a more generic instrument. C. T. Beck (1995) designed the Postpartum Depression Checklist (PDC) based on findings of two qualitative studies with postpartum women. It is a practical tool for eliciting a woman's feelings about her experiences. When a standardized interview is desired, these specific tools are recommended.

O'Hara and colleagues (O'Hara et al., 1992) have developed an instrument to assess social-role adjustment in childbearing women, the Postpartum Adjustment Questionnaire (PPAQ). The PPAQ allows assessment of a woman's functioning in roles likely related to postpartum distress, including worker, friend, mother, and wife.

Clinical Interview. In clinical assessment of new mothers, the interviewer needs to attend to each of the risk factors mentioned previously. The order in which this is done can enhance or inhibit the therapeutic alliance. Given the stigma of postpartum distress, most new mothers are extremely sensitive to any hint that their current symptoms represent a failing on their part. The wise examiner will postpone discussion of early childhood experiences or previous personal difficulties until rapport is established, and even then treat these issues with extreme care. Beginning the assessment by focusing on the current symptoms makes the new mother feel supported and understood. What she really wants to do is find some quick relief for the pain she is suffering. The therapist can validate her feelings by first focusing on her day-to-day life. Issues from her past or her current relationships may certainly be important to her recovery, but she cannot attend to those issues if she is getting only 2 hours of sleep per night, crying every day, or having frightening panic attacks. Treatment and evaluation are closely linked at this point, since giving the new mother even one helpful idea to put into practice immediately, with some effect on her symptoms, conveys to her that therapy is really valuable. In the words of Hickman (1994), first "put out the fire" before expecting to accomplish any other changes. Gruen (1993) validates this point.

In the initial evaluation, the examiner needs to get the nitty-gritty details of the new mother's symptoms. Ask for specifics about her sleeping, eating, crying, details of her days, and where her time goes. It is necessary to ask, in a very forthright but reassuring manner, about any scary thoughts or anxieties. Most women will not confide the thoughts common to postpartum OCD unless they are asked explicitly. Establish the course of her symptoms since the birth, especially changes in symptoms. Throughout this exploration, begin to integrate intervention with the assessment, offering education, validation, and reassurance about the woman's symptoms. This is particularly important with OCD; these women relax noticeably when reassured that there is little possibility of acting on the thoughts. Having this knowledge and sharing it conveys that the therapist is a person who understands and can be helpful with the woman's postpartum distress, enhancing the therapeutic alliance.

After a thorough understanding of the postpartum symptom picture is achieved, the examiner can explore immediate history. Beginning with the physical history removes the onus of guilt, validating that much of the distress that the woman is experiencing is related to physical and emotional changes of pregnancy, labor, birth, and the postpartum. Assess the course of the pregnancy, labor, and birth, including any complications. Complications are important physically, as in Sheehan's syndrome, as well as emotionally. The new mother's interpretation of the events of labor and birth is important, and provides clues about her view of her world and her ability to control it. Ask about whether she is breast feeding, or has discontinued. If so, why, and how does she feel about it? When this immediate medical history is complete, assess previous medical history. Focus on her general health, especially her history of previous hormonal or gynecological difficulties, that is, premenstrual syndrome (PMS), infertility, irregular periods, pregnancy loss, or abortion. What medications and substances does she use routinely, therapeutic or recreational drugs, nicotine, caffeine, or vitamin and mineral supplements? How are her eating habits, and is there a history of eating disorder? Are there any medical conditions in her family, such as thyroid abnormalities? Is there any family or personal history of emotional problems? If discussion of history is kept brief, it is less likely to put her on the defensive. The examiner then focuses on the current psychosocial situation, including changes, losses, and stressors. How does her experience with this new baby match her expectations? What is her previous experience with children/infants? Assess her work situation, ask about maternity leave and her feelings about returning to work. Who comprises her support system, and does she have people to call for support or information in her religious community or family? How does she take care of herself (i.e., fun, exercise, naps, friends)? At this point, rapport may permit in-depth discussion of family background, including issues reactivated by the birth. Gather this information without sending the message that history is of primary importance, because to the new mother, her current situation is what impacts her most strongly.

Attend to the relationship with the baby and other children. It may be easier for the new mother to talk about the relationship with the baby first, exploring her feelings toward the child and herself as a parent. Inquire about this child's temperament and fit with her expectations. Does she feel like the baby is hers? Significant sources of stress exist for her if she feels inadequate or disliked by her baby. This is extremely critical and requires specific intervention if the relationship is not going well. Having the infant present for at least part of the session is valuable, to watch for clues to the attachment. Observe her confidence in handling the baby, her responsivity, and her eye contact with the baby. Practitioners need an understanding of normal expectations for infant-parent interactions; see Field (1987); Field et al. (1990, 1991); and Pickens and Field (1993).

Assessing the status of the marital or partner relationship is critical for social support as well as increased risk. Including her partner in one of the initial assessment sessions can provide an opportunity to evaluate the relationship and its role in her postpartum distress. While for some couples marital discord may precede postpartum distress, for others the postpartum emotions are negatively impacting the relationship. It is necessary to clarify this as early as possible, for the status of the relationship can greatly affect the new mother's individual progress. Once the direction of influence is clear, treatment can be planned accordingly. If the issues are primarily individual, the spouse may be brought in from time to time to support her. Or the focus of treatment may need to be on the relationship.

The examiner needs to ask about how having a baby has changed things for the couple. If they seem open, the examiner can pursue the issue further, asking about conflict and their ability to resolve it. Is her partner providing emotional as well as practical support? The partner may be extremely helpful and understanding, carrying much of the household and childcare burden while maintaining the family income. At other times, the spouse feels that the new mom is malingering, or focusing on the negative. New mothers often report that the husband thinks she should "just smile," or "pull herself up by her bootstraps." These messages produce more guilt in the new mother; she feels her partner is saying that if she were just stronger, she would not be having these difficulties. Getting these kinds of messages out in the open represents an intervention; the therapist can educate the couple, validate the mother's feelings, and stress the need to work through the negative feelings, rather than just "act happy."

Assess how the partner is holding up with the current situation. If the partner is shouldering the bulk of the family responsibilities, the partner may need support and a chance to vent as well. Many partners become frustrated and distressed themselves with their inability to "solve" the new mother's problems. Offering support and education to the spouse helps the partner continue this vital assistance. While this part of the assessment takes place, observation of the couple's dynamics, communication style, and skills gives valuable information. It is important again to keep the focus on the new mother's difficulties, solving those first and foremost. To turn the assessment session into a relationship therapy session, without that being the couple's explicit wish, may alienate one or both members of the dyad and be detrimental to the therapeutic relationship with the woman. Finally, this dyadic session can give insight into the partner's view on the new mother's recovery. The spouse may be very hopeful, willing to have her in therapy. Or therapy and/or medication may be viewed negatively, with the partner feeling that the new mother should be able to solve problems such as these within the family.

Finally, the examiner needs to ask what steps the new mother and/or couple have taken to cope with her distress. Have they consulted other professionals, tried medication, or worked on the mother taking breaks? It is important to know what they have already been through in order to (a) correct any misperceptions that have developed in contact with misinformed professionals; (b) avoid duplicating their efforts to date; and (c) applaud them for their persistence. When all of this information has been gathered, explain the therapist's view of the situation to the new mother and, if possible, her partner. Highlight the resources they have available, with lots of compliments for what they have managed to date. The risk factors in their situation are summarized, so that they can see what is essential to address in the therapy. This relieves much of the guilt for the new mother and the couple, as they see the contributions to the postpartum distress which are (a) normal and (b) beyond what they can control. The treatment plan is discussed, detailing individual, marital, or group therapy, or medication consultation. By the end of the evaluation, the therapist can forge a treatment contract, outlining the number of sessions and examples of interventions. The new mother and her partner have been educated about postpartum distress, its causes, and that it is treatable. They leave in a hopeful state.

Assessment Example

Ginger was a 34-year-old married mother of a 2-month-old baby. Her new husband had been transferred and the day after they returned from their honeymoon they moved across the country away from Ginger's home state. They had been married for 5 months when Ginger became pregnant. Ginger had always been independent; she had worked in a managerial position before marriage, had owned a home, and had traveled extensively. In the new city, Ginger knew no one. Pregnancy had been difficult; a threatened miscarriage, partial bedrest, and infections sapped her strength. Previously, she had been extremely healthy, both physically and emotionally. There was no family history of psychiatric difficulty or thyroid dysfunction. She experienced a stressful vaginal birth; she lost three pints of blood and there was a knot in the umbilical cord. Other than fatigue, Ginger denied unresolved feelings about the birth. She was having great trouble returning to sleep after the baby woke for night feedings. She just lay in bed, feeling too tired to sleep. Ginger was eating adequately, and resting each day for about an hour, but she was crying about 3 hours each day. She denied specific worries or obsessions; she was not suicidal or homicidal. Her social isolation was intense; other than two neighbors, she had contact with only her husband and the baby. Ginger missed her family a great deal and none of her relatives had visited the baby. Her husband had a 1-hour commute each way to his job, and was extremely tired when he returned home. He helped with one night feeding, and cared for the baby briefly on weekends, but did little else with the baby. Ginger said he was always tired, and she was reluctant to ask him to do much. But she herself got no breaks. He played golf each weekend, went fishing every other week, and traveled overnight about 3 times per month. The couple had been out to dinner the previous weekend, a welcome break. They were not in much conflict, but the relationship sounded strained and empty in Ginger's description. Ginger was blaming herself for her feelings of depression and fatigue. Having a family and being married had been her desire; she echoed the familiar "Something must be the matter with me." She loved the baby; he was easy and slept well. She had talked to her obstetrician about her feelings, and the doctor had offered to give her an antidepressant and sleeping pills. But Ginger refused because she was breast feeding.

Ginger was undergoing a normal postpartum adjustment complicated by several factors. She was socially isolated. She was grieving the loss of her family, home, and former independent lifestyle. The marriage had gone from the honeymoon stage almost immediately to parenthood, with little time for adjustment. The couple had not established solid communication skills when the baby came along. Failed expectations were causing Ginger to question whether getting married and having this baby had been mistakes. Her husband was stressed by his new job, his sudden family, and this transformation in his wife. Ginger had been a caretaker in her family, and did not see her own needs as important. Ginger was not adept at conveying to her family that she needed their contact and support, even long-distance.

The treatment plan involved individual, group, and marital therapy sessions. Group therapy allowed Ginger to connect with other women, receiving validation for her distress and her lack of blame. Individual sessions focused on giving her permission to take care of herself. She wrote some letters and let her family know that she needed them, and they responded favorably. Marital sessions gave the couple a chance to improve communication skills and negotiate roles in their still-new relationship.

PSYCHOTHERAPY INTERVENTIONS

Individual Therapy. There is scant literature addressing the process of individual therapy with postpartum women. One exception addresses the utilization of interpersonal psychotherapy (IPT; Klerman et al., 1984) with postpartum depression (O'Hara, 1996; Stuart & O'Hara, 1995). These researchers propose that postpartum depression arises in a context of biological vulnerability and social disruptions. Interpersonal psychotherapy is well-suited for postpartum depression because of the importance of interpersonal relationships in this time period and the emphasis of IPT on role transitions. The initial controlled treatment trial of 12 sessions of IPT appeared to be effective for postpartum women in this sample (O'Hara, 1996). The therapy in this study focused on the relationship with the baby, the relationship with partner, and the transition back to work.

The approach to individual therapy described here combines this interpersonal focus with active incorporation of cognitive-behavioral techniques. The new mother's most intense need, when presenting for therapy, is control and decrease of the symptoms which overwhelm her and interfere with her functioning. Postpartum women need to achieve some relief of these symptoms first and foremost. Understanding the source of feelings may be helpful, but she needs to take action to feel better and act differently, which McGrath (1992) describes as "action therapy." At the same time, new mothers need to address their feelings about having a postpartum disorder. Dysphoric distress, intrusive thoughts, or panic attacks create guilt in the new mother. She blames herself. This is probably her first experience with emotions or behavior that requires professional intervention, and she needs to resolve the guilt and fault she aims at herself. Telling her story is very healing (Azar, 1994). She may need to grieve the loss of the ideal postpartum adjustment she envisioned. Having a new baby was not supposed to be like this, and she will need to sort out her feelings and come to an understanding of "why" that she can live with. If these two needs are ignored or bypassed by health professionals working with the new mother, the therapeutic relationship may be compromised. The goal is to help her establish some stability, and move on to address family-of-origin or other background issues only if and when she is ready.

The beginning of individual therapy involves education and validation. She can be given materials to read about postpartum disorders. The therapist can reassure her that she is not crazy, weak, or a failure. Tell her that she is going through a very real developmental crisis, and intense feelings and changes in roles and relationships are part of that adjustment. Help her recognize the multiple stressors that have gotten her to this point, from biological and biochemical changes to societal expectations, so she can realize that *it is not her fault*. Statistics about the prevalence of her particular disorder and contact with other women who have experienced similar problems are helpful, so she can see that *she is not alone*. Finally, she needs reassurance that she will get better. To give a realistic picture of the course of treatment, she needs to hear that postpartum recovery is an up-and-down process, with a normal course of good days and bad days. Many postpartum women have felt devastated, after several good days or weeks, to find their symptoms back in full force. When this happens, the woman inevitably feels hopeless, that she will never be normal again. This is not true; she has not lost all progress when a setback occurs. This setback often comes just when her menstrual cycle is about to resume; an upset in hormones may trigger the setback. Practically, there are many ways to get this information across to her. Handouts, pamphlets, books, and articles can be provided to educate the new mother and her family, such as Dunnewold and Sanford (1994) and Dix (1985). Postpartum Support International and Depression After Delivery (see Table 1, p. 8) can provide peer support via telephone, as well as worthwhile articles and pamphlets.

Providing tools for symptom relief is just as important a priority. New mothers thrive on concrete, behavioral strategies to feel better. They have little time available to take care of their own needs, and need efficient strategies that show quick results. Initially, the therapist can help the woman determine which symptoms are most pressing or distressing. Rank order symptoms, and decide which should be tackled first. Physical symptoms such as problems with eating and sleeping must be alleviated before she can look at other issues. She cannot meet new people to develop a support system if she is not sleeping at night.

Core strategies for treatment of postpartum distress are physical and emotional self-care, social support, and structure. These strategies impact many problems, and are helpful with most women. The first strategy employed is to help the mother plan her physical self-care, as outlined in Dunnewold and Sanford (1994). She needs permission from the therapist to take care of herself if she is to have enough emotional and physical energy to nurture this baby, let alone other family members. What changes are needed to ensure she gets enough rest, eats right, and exercises? In the working world, breaks are the law. But new mothers taking care of newborns all day rarely manage this necessity, even though breaks are a vital part of having enough energy to keep up with their responsibilities. Help the new mother plan for when, and how, she will take breaks. She needs 5 minutes to relax every morning, afternoon, and evening. Perhaps she can read one page of the newspaper, or listen to some special music while she has a glass of juice, putting her feet up. Mothers who are working outside the home need breaks from baby care other than their time at work. No one can do a job nonstop without time off every day.

Physical self-care is intricately connected to the next strategy, developing (or utilizing) a support system, as the therapist and client identify who can help with infant care or household tasks. This work involves values clarification and time management. Is a clean house really the priority, or is it better to spend time holding the baby? Many new mothers, used to relying on their own resources, need to be encouraged to reach out and ask for help. She may know lots of people, but is accustomed to appearing strong and managing on her own. It may be a challenge to ask others, including her partner, for assistance. Besides practical help, the new mother needs people in the same life stage to talk with at least once a week. The therapist working with postpartum women needs familiarity with resources for new parents in the community, such as postpartum support groups, postpartum exercise classes, or a group devoted to learning about infant development. Take an active role in helping her identify these resources in her own neighborhood or religious communities. Help her structure time to be with people. She can call a friend or invite them for a walk, to a class on parenting, or for a coffee break.

Structure is the third strategy involved in successful treatment of postpartum women. Because she is overwhelmed, she needs concrete detail from the therapist on how to structure her life. Begin by working out a daily schedule of when to rest or nap, and what to eat. Because of the changeability of most infants' schedules, this must be flexible, such as "call friend in the morning" or "take break after baby's bath." Structure is useful in giving her some control over her life, and getting her to focus on her own physical and emotional needs. Structure is employed in dealing with most issues and concerns postpartum. In the following sections, additional strategies for dealing with some of these issues are detailed, as well as elaboration on the use of structure.

Physical Symptoms. Underlying medical causes for physical symptoms need to be ruled out with an in-depth physical examination. Thyroid dysfunction or other hormonal problems need to be ruled out. If the woman has a clean bill of health from her physician, physical symptoms may continue to be related to the levels of stress in her life. Attention needs to be paid to the mother's exercise and diet, as well as emotional self-care such as having fun and taking breaks. Six small meals a day can help keep blood sugar up, stabilizing mood (Dalton, 1993). She may have cravings or lack appetite. With cravings, reasonable portions may be allowed rather than denial, which tends to make the urge worse. If she lacks appetite, she can identify "comfort foods" which she ate during childhood or in happy times.

Many new mothers are fatigued and reassurance about the reality of that feeling when caring for a newborn may help. Many women have difficulty returning to sleep after feeding the baby at night. Be sure that intake of caffeine (Bruce et al., 1992) or alcohol is not the cause. Intake of calcium and magnesium supplements may be helpful with many women (Pearlstein, 1993). Worries may be the culprit; behavioral strategies such as journaling and thought-stopping can help. Distinguish between worry about daily concerns and caring for the baby from worry about sleep itself (Watts, Coyle, & East, 1994), and plan treatment accordingly. As the new mother loses more and more sleep, her anxiety rises about functioning in her sleep-deprived state. To interrupt this vicious cycle, sleep hygiene is effective (Morin et al., 1994). Clients retrain their bodies to relax at bedtime by following a regular schedule: avoiding naps, sleep-disruptive drugs or stimulants, and heavy meals or hunger near bedtime; employing a relaxing evening routine; and avoiding lying in bed awake or using bed for activities other than sleep. Visual imagery and relaxation training are valuable tools, too.

Hyperventilation, dizziness, shaking, hot or cold flashes, numbness or tingling, and heart palpitations can all be signs of a panic attack, and should be treated accordingly with behavioral intervention and/or medication (Clum & Surls, 1993). Psychological coping strategies such as relaxation training, cognitive restructuring, distraction, exposure, and flooding are all effective with panic attacks. Eliminating caffeine from her diet is necessary as well (Bruce et al., 1992). The woman needs to be told that these are just symptoms or reactions in her body related to biochemical changes, and they have no meaning other than that she is anxious. She is not going to die, or go crazy. She can use self-talk, relaxation, and distraction to focus her attention more positively. If she can identify a specific traumatic event as a trigger, a program of progressive desensitization may be indicated. The therapist can help her identify the events which lead to her panic, and teach both cognitive restructuring and relaxation for coping. Bibliotherapy may be useful; Wilson (1986) and Bourne (1990) offer two of the best works.

Stomach pain and butterflies in the stomach may be related to OCD (Sichel, 1990). Physical soreness, headaches, and constipation or diarrhea may all be stress-related, and thus may resolve as the woman tackles the stresses in her life.

Feelings. New mothers face a range of powerful feelings, from joy to anger to dysphoria. She may have intense anxiety, sadness, guilt, and feelings of loss. Feelings of inadequacy, being overwhelmed, and lacking in confidence are also problematic. Therapeutic intervention with the new mother for these feelings is a process of (a) acknowledging and expressing the feelings; (b) accepting the feelings through reassurance from others and positive self-talk; and (c) problem-solving on the issue, to see if changes can be made which will relieve the feelings. The validation in item (b) is necessary not just from the therapist, but from the partner or other persons close to the postpartum woman. These steps apply to most postpartum feelings, and are fully explained below. To balance this focus on the negative, the new mother needs to structure similar amounts of time to attend to positive feelings. She needs to be told to look for and even write down her positive feelings and accomplishments. This will reassure her that her life is not all negative.

The first step in dealing with any of these negative feelings is to support and encourage her to express and accept them. Her life has changed, irrevocably. Let her know it is acceptable to feel sad, angry, or overwhelmed when adjusting to a new baby. Listen to her feelings of loss, lack of control, or guilt. This was an effective intervention in a study cited by Holden (1991). Reassure her that she is still an OK person even if she does not feel wonderful about this new part of her life. The new mother may need direction on how to express and accept these feelings. Structure is again worthwhile. Setting aside even 10 minutes a day to cry, or write in a journal, or talk sad feelings into a tape recorder, or scream out her angry feelings while in the shower, can give her much needed relief. She needs to name her anger, sadness, and loss. Many women will argue that they do not want to focus on these feelings; avoidance is preferred. Reframe the time structured for focusing on the feelings as more efficient, therefore it will free her energy for other pursuits. If she fights her sadness all day, she uses up a tremendous amount of energy. If she spends some concentrated time on the feeling, rather than fighting it, she will be working toward resolution and she will feel better. She may have to agree to a trial period of several days before she sees the value. In structuring time to attend to the feeling, it is important too that she have a strategy planned for switching gears when the scheduled time is over. Have her set the timer, and when it rings, she performs the preplanned activity. This works best if it is an active distraction, such as taking a walk, calling a support person, or taking a shower. She then feels in control of the feeling, instead of it controlling her.

Along with expressing these feelings, and telling herself that they are understandable, she may need the therapist to take her through a problem-solving process. If specific issues are behind the feelings, can she change them? Of course she cannot change that she had a girl when she wanted a boy, but perhaps she can change that her partner does not seem involved with the baby. With issues that cannot be changed, she may need to grieve that loss, acknowledging it and structuring time to focus on the loss and related feelings. This is needed when there has been some other loss in the new mother's life, such as a death, an illness, or a move. She needs permission to grieve both concrete or less obvious losses, such as her lifestyle.

For the postpartum woman, anger may be the most surprising emotion. The anger wells up, inducing guilt. She wonders what she could possibly have to feel angry about. Anger during this life transition is legitimate, and most of it has to do with expectations. She needs to hear she is normal for feeling angry when she did not expect to feel so upset or tired, or for the baby to cry all the time, or to look like her least favorite relative. She needs a safe, nondestructive outlet for her anger. Some women prefer active methods to let their anger out, such as exercise, punching a pillow, or screaming. Others do better with journaling, meditation, or imagery about letting the anger drift away. She can make a list of what works for her, and keep it on the refrigerator or her desk to refer to in angry moments. Assertive communication skills can be used in voicing anger to others, for example, "I" messages and behavioral descriptions.

The new mother often feels overwhelmed; she feels little control in her life. Help her identify one part of her life over which she does have control. The therapist can advise her to write this one thing down, reviewing it to reassure herself that she can finish tasks. Assist her in picking one task that she will attempt to complete each day, such as keeping one area of the house picked up. It can be extremely comforting to list everything that she does do in one day: how many times she fed, diapered, burped, walked, or dressed the baby. Filling a sheet of paper with this data gives her a palpable record. Besides validating the important task of infant care, it shows in a concrete manner that she is achieving a lot. She can add one task every several days, building slowly to avoid that overwhelming feeling that there is too much to be done. Help her review what she has finished, rather than focus on what is left undone.

Most parents experience guilt from time to time, because of the demands of balancing personal needs, work demands, and child care tasks. Schedules and structure are immensely helpful, allotting time for everyone's needs. She may find it helpful to use a kitchen timer to play with the baby for a few minutes, then take equal time for herself, then do a household chore. While this feels artificial at first, it can increase her sense of control. Positive self-talk and realistic expectations need to be initiated to deal with guilt, too; she again needs to see what she has done, not what is left undone.

To battle a lack of confidence or feelings of inadequacy in the new mother, debunk the idea that *anyone* automatically feels like a parent. Parental instinct is a myth; comfort with parenting is based on previous experience, and grows with time. Stating this is tremendously reassuring. Encourage the new mother to identify ways she feels confident, or to get instruction in childcare if necessary. Have the new mother write "I can be a good enough parent" on paper and post it around to remind herself, or review it daily. Reinforce that everyone must develop their own parenting style, and there is no one right way to be a parent. The woman may be comparing herself to friends, siblings, or reference books, finding herself sorely lacking. Discuss what she thinks is important as a parent, and help her identify concrete tasks she might undertake that would put her philosophy into practice.

Fluctuating hormones, fatigue, and the uncertainty of taking on a new role all contribute to the sensitivity new mothers often report. Determine when she is most sensitive or irritable. Is she most likely to feel hurt when she is tired, hungry, or feeling isolated? If a pattern emerges, work to eliminate the triggers. Nurturing her sense of humor can decrease her irritability. She needs to try to laugh daily, whether at herself, her situation, or something outside of all this. Giving her an assignment to "laugh or have fun twice a day" can fill this need in the new mother.

This hypersensitivity may be exacerbated by miscommunication. For example, Mary's spouse came home, going straight to play with the baby, without even a hello. Mary felt neglected and hurt each time. When she spoke up and asked for a greeting, her partner did so each day before rushing to see the baby. Many new mothers project criticism into the words of significant others. In Joan's case, her partner came home two times and exclaimed "You are still in your nightgown!" Rather than running off in tears, the therapist encouraged her to take deep breaths and ask "What do you mean by that?" the next time it happened. Her partner reported worrying about her, but not criticizing her, as Joan had assumed.

Anxiety and worry are the most common feelings of new parents. Explore the nature of the new mother's worries. The therapist needs to ask directly about any obsessive thoughts, and whether she has envisioned harm coming to her baby. It is critical to differentiate the thoughts of OCD from the delusions of psychosis. If it is clear that the thoughts are ego dystonic, reassure her about her baby's safety and the normalcy of these worries. If there are situations which increase her worries or obsessions, such as watching the news on TV or reading the newspaper, she may need to decrease these activities for a while.

Behavioral strategies are effective with these postpartum worries, whether obsessive in nature or not. Structure a "worry time" each day. She can keep a notebook handy, jotting down her worries through the day to save until the appointed time. As she records the worry, she really should think it through rather than work to suppress it. Once recorded and saved for "worry time," she can use distraction to get through to that time. This is consistent with the work of Salkovskis and P. Campbell (1994) and Roemer and Borkovec (1994), that suppressing thoughts results in increased intrusion. When "worry time" arrives, she should get out the notebook and worry about her concerns for 20 minutes. This represents revised habituation, an effective treatment for OCD (Roth & Church, 1994). When the time is up, an activity to switch gears is essential. Writing worries on an erasable board and erasing them, or on paper and tearing them up, or wearing a fat rubber band on her wrist to snap as a stimulus for thought-stopping can be effective. Visual imagery, switching channels on an envisioned TV screen, is also helpful for some women. Relaxation skills can be taught and employed to deal with these anxieties (Halonen & Passman, 1985).

Cognitive therapy is valuable in the treatment of worries and obsessions. Acceptance of the worries usually comes if she believes she can still be a good-enough parent in spite of them. Encourage her to recognize that they are just thoughts, and she is not likely to act upon them. Reassure her that she knows the thoughts are wrong, she does not want to act upon them, and she has no history suggesting that she will be violent. Evaluating the probability of risk may help, as she sees that the risk is quite low (Van Oppen & Arntz, 1994). Focus on her responsibility in other realms; she *is* taking good care of her child. Intrinsic in helping her deal with the obsessions may be the issue of control. These worries or obsessions may reflect her awareness that she does not have total control, and cannot perfectly protect her child from harm in this world. Just voicing this may be freeing, as she sees that no one can perfectly protect their child. Using coping self-talk, she tells herself that she is taking all reasonable precautions, and this is all she can do to protect her child. An effective reframing is that she can see the danger and take extra precautions because she is exquisitely sensitive. Caution is advised, for overprotective mothers may take this to the extreme. This intervention is likely useful only with mothers who have these worries, but have not altered their behavior toward their infant as a result.

Beliefs and Cognitions. Postpartum women often have ideas which compound their distress. Cognitive therapy is effective with these negative thought patterns, but action strategies are important too. Tackling these maladaptive thoughts begins with realistic expectations. Expectations of total control and perfectionism often plague new mothers. The new mother needs reassurance that this is normal, even though it is a huge change from her prebaby life. The therapist can help her fine tune her expectations, finding where she does have control, and define reasonable, achievable goals. Flexible structure for her day helps to achieve balance in life once again.

Positive self-talk, reviewing where she does have control, and reminding herself that it is tolerable and normal *not* to control everything, is again a useful intervention. Giving the assignment to purposely make harmless mistakes may enable her to relax. She may not realize that imperfection is survivable unless she "goofs." Often it is easiest to pick small things, such as putting the baby's shirt on backwards or leaving the dirty dishes in the sink overnight.

Cognitions about perfection and control are often centered on body image. For the postpartum woman who feels like her body is foreign, dressing in the morning may trigger lots of self-deprecating talk. Taking time for exercise and healthful diet is important. Postpartum exercise classes can give her a sense of tackling the problem, within a socially supportive setting. Resuming any physical activity that she enjoyed in the past helps her regain control of her body. Negative self-talk can be replaced with coping self-talk. The therapist can urge her to find one feature about her body that she likes, and focus on that, adding one feature to accept each week. She may need to grieve the loss of her prebaby body, for in some ways she will never be the same. Social support, such as Overeaters Anonymous and Weight Watchers, may fit for individual women.

Questions about self-esteem and identity are common after the birth of a baby. The new mother may need to discuss her former self, and how she can integrate this with a new identity as a parent. The therapist can help her formulate concrete ways to put the qualities she desires into practice, or to recognize how she is achieving this persona.

Pam had always considered herself to be an intellectually oriented person. Caring for a newborn all day, she did not feel smart or informed at all. The therapist pointed out that she was reading all the baby books she could get her hands on, and had transferred her skills, temporarily, to this arena. Reassured, she capitalized on it by joining a mother's group which reviewed the latest childcare books for each other.

Much self-doubt in early parenthood can be traced to the switch from activities, usually paid, in which the mother received regular feedback on her performance, to the daily grind of infant care without feedback. Babies do not look up at their mothers and say "Thanks, Mom, good job." Concrete rewards are few for the difficult, immensely valuable job of raising children. Acknowledge this void, and help the postpartum woman plan ways to reward herself or ask for feedback from others. Have her list strengths, as a parent or otherwise, and review them each day. She can use positive self-talk to tally her accomplishments, and then relate these to her partner, asking for reinforcement of her contributions to the family. Pediatricians offer feedback on parenting, with evidence from the baby's weight gain or developmental milestones. To build confidence in parenting, the mother may want to take a parenting class.

The new mother's identity in other areas deserves nurturing through devoting time to other interests. She can set aside time to renew an old interest or develop a new one. Having the therapist draw a pie chart of the various roles in her life is reassuring. She is a mother, wife, worker, dancer, daughter, and friend. Care of a newborn consumes the whole pie at first. Setting aside time and energy to revive those other parts of her self can be valuable.

Confusion is common after the birth of a baby because of sleep deprivation and new responsibilities, especially when coupled with fluctuating hormones. Reassurance, stress management, and decreasing expectations are important. Making lists, self-talk, and verbal rehearsal can help the new mother stay focused on the task at hand. Address any clinical issues that interfere with her ability to concentrate.

Marital/Family Therapy. Careful assessment determines which came first: relationship discord or postpartum distress. If postpartum distress is conceptualized as an adjustment disorder, then a primary goal of treatment will be helping the couple adjust to the changes in their relationship that result from this new developmental crisis (Whiffen,1992). Research has repeatedly suggested that these normal marital adjustments after the birth of a baby may be even more difficult for the depressed woman (O'Hara et al., 1990). Even if the relationship seems unaffected, the partner can provide significant support in the woman's recovery (Gruen, 1993). Family-of-origin relationships often must be addressed, for they may not have impacted the new mother in a healthy way.

Couples Therapy. As with individual therapy, couples treatment begins with education, validation, and normalization. New parents relax when told that the adjustment to a new baby, even when not the first, is a time of stress, and mixed feelings are expected. Cultural expectations lead them to worry about what might be wrong with them for having conflict at this allegedly wonderful time. Removing this blame helps the couple revise expectations to appropriate levels, easing the transition to parenthood (Kalmuss et al., 1992). Having planned in advance how they would divide family responsibilities, the couple may be dismayed to see they are duplicating their families-of-origin. Reassuring them that, under stress, many individuals revert to the powerful models they witnessed growing up can relieve guilt. This is not only natural but revocable. With the therapist's guidance, they can resume the patterns of relating established before the birth. Teaching conflict management and communication skills is essential, especially if marital discord precedes the birth. Couples need to be taught not to withdraw during conflict, to take breaks before the conflict escalates, and to avoid insults. They need to be educated in using

"I" messages and descriptions of behavior rather than attacks against the person. Recent research indicates that increasing positive interaction in the couple may be most critical (Gottman, 1993; Markman & Notarius 1994). Works by these authors suggest that positive must outweigh negative in marriages by a ratio of 5 to 1 for those marriages to be healthy. Couples' resources for developing these skills are McKay and Mitchell (1995); McKay, Fanning, and Paleg (1994), and Markman and Notarius (1994).

New parents tend to focus on the baby to the exclusion of their partner. Spurred on by the new financial demands, partners may increase their work commitments. Mothers often have greater involvement with the baby, because of breast feeding or extended leave for newborn care. The stress of one partner being absent, neglected, or uninvolved creates resentment and further stress. The mother needs to see her role in taking it all on, and her partner needs to be challenged to see any insecurity about the role in letting her do so. Structuring family life works to alleviate this imbalance. Talking with the couple about how they would like to divide household and childcare jobs — making lists of responsibilities — opens up communication about these issues. Having the couple set up a weekly "date," in the home or out, can make them feel more connected. Daily time to make contact, whether sharing notes from their days or sitting together physically simply holding hands, is crucial. Making this a priority is critical if they are to preserve their relationship as a couple, not just two people parenting together. Couples tend to think in terms of grand plans, evenings out, or weekends off without the baby. Smaller amounts of positive time focused on each other are equally important. Encouraging them to have more fun together and to explicitly express more affection and appreciation can be valuable in improving the relationship.

Assigning the less-involved partner specific childcare tasks can increase involvement with the baby. While many new mothers are protective of their role with the baby, and may prefer to have the other parent tackle the dishes rather than the bath, it is helpful to point out that the child's relationship with both parents is important. The more-involved parent can "disappear," running an errand or taking a walk, so the less-involved parent can find his or her own way with the baby. Nothing interferes with a partner feeling comfortable with a childcare task more than a hovering mother offering advice on the "right" way to burp the baby.

Negotiating values differences may be a critical role for the therapist to take up with the couple. One parent may want to raise the child one way, while the other parent feels this would be a major mistake. Sometimes a trade-off system works: one parent can decide about the child's eating while the other decides about the toys. Helping parents recognize their individual strengths in terms of parenting contributes to this process. One may be more organized, while the other is more spontaneous. The therapist can point out that they balance each other, and can maximize their strengths in this new role if they negotiate first. Giving them concrete strategies like counting to 10 or scheduling times for such discussions may be necessary.

The therapist may need to initiate discussion of how the partner contributes to the new mother's self-care. The new mom may be reluctant to ask the partner for help. She often states that "My partner has worked all day." The partner can be encouraged to offer help, which he or she may be reluctant to do for fear of implying that the new mom is doing an inadequate job. If the parent working outside the home takes 20 minutes to unwind each evening before arriving home, he or she may be more willing to take over with the baby upon walking in the door. The mother may be able to give her partner this down time if they negotiate it in advance, and then take a much-deserved soak in the tub or walk around the block. Having the partner in charge of a certain evening or afternoon every week gives the mother a regular respite while giving that partner a chance to find the best way to relate to the child.

Couple sessions may be necessary to address obstacles to treatment from the partner. Many individuals still focus on an independent mode of dealing with crisis; the partner may want the spouse to "be strong" and "solve this problem within the family" rather than through outside support and intervention. The partner may be opposed to the new mother taking medication. To overcome resistance, have the couple attend a session together and learn about the biochemical changes which may have tipped the balance in the current difficulties. Normalizing the situation and reassuring both that she is not crazy or weak can engage the partner's full support of her treatment.

Couple sessions also serve as a forum for the partner's own stresses. The partner may need a place to voice hopelessness, frustration, and confusion about what has gone wrong and why it could not be stopped. The partner is working, caring for the mother and the infant, and taking care of the house; caretaker burn-out may be likely. Support and validation are offered in the couple sessions, encouraging the partner to take care of personal needs. The partner needs an evening out with friends, regular exercise, rest, healthful diet, and even a place to voice frustrations with the mother's symptoms. Recognizing the partner's contributions and needs fosters the therapeutic alliance.

The Mother-Child Relationship. The relationship with the baby can be a source of stress, support, or both to the new mother. Knowing that the attachment process is slow and gradual, rather than instantaneous at birth, is reassuring for many new mothers. The baby may be the focus of the new mother's feelings, from anger to protectiveness to joy. The new mother needs to hear reassuring words from the therapist about the range of feelings that this closeness creates; it is normal to feel frustrated, angry, and protective, as well as joyful and loving. Cramer (1993) hypothesized that postpartum depression is a disturbance in the attachment relationship, though there is no controlled research evidence to support this theory. Clinically, problems with the mother-baby bond do appear in some women with postpartum distress, but this is not universal. Nevertheless, the mother-infant relationship does need to be addressed when a mother is experiencing postpartum distress because of the far-reaching effects on the baby. Many depressed mothers worry about this and they need to be reassured that their relationships with their babies are tempered by many other factors, including each baby's temperament and the mother's relationships with other adults.

Observing mother-infant interaction in the clinical setting is a powerful start. The therapist offers reassurance about how well the interaction is going, or reinforces positive behaviors. If this cannot be arranged in the office, the mother or another party may videotape the interaction at home. The therapist can watch the tape and give the mother feedback on her behavior with the baby. Give the mother some positive comments, such as "See how she smiles at you" and "She turns when she hears your voice," while providing instruction on improving interaction with the baby. Compliments such as these let the mother know she is on the right track. Her anxiety decreases, enabling her to be more responsive to the baby. Concrete teaching about ways to play with the baby may be needed, teaching the mother to mirror, respond vocally to the baby, or get the baby's attention (Pickens & Field, 1993). This can be done in session, or the mother can find information in books: Lansky (1993) and Munger and Bowden (1993) provide valuable resources. Setting up times to play with the baby, or to observe the baby and assess his or her abilities can be effective.

With the changing of the family structure, changes in feelings for all family members, including other children, occur. Mothers of older children frequently feel guilt about how the new baby has altered the older child's life. She may feel anger at the older child, who is more independent, verbal, and able to challenge her as a parent. These feelings can be normalized. Time devoted to special activities, playing, or reading with the older child, eases the guilt and fosters that relationship. Playing "baby," allowing the older child to pretend to be a baby and drink from a bottle, rock, play with a rattle, and so forth, diffuses sibling rivalry and allows the mother to nurture the child. Even latency age boys will "play baby," even though they might reject these attempts at nurturing by their mother if they are not "pretend."

Family-of-Origin Issues. This life transition may create stresses on the relationship with either parents' family-of-origin. Telling the history helps the new parent realize the connection between the family and adjustment to parenthood. Boundaries may need to be reinforced; what is the role of parents versus grandparents? Unresolved issues often need to be addressed, or grieved if the adult has made a realistic effort and the situation remains unchanged. A problem-solving strategy is recommended, defining what she or he would like to have different with the extended family, and planning specific steps to that goal. Family sessions may be indicated, or writing letters to family members may suffice. The therapist can review drafts of letters for wording, enabling the new parent to voice feelings and/or requests in a productive manner. Writing a script and rehearsing it in session or in front of a mirror are good preparations for talking to family members. Gestalt "empty chair" technique is useful in processing these feelings. New parents may want to change their relationships with families-of-origin, but are reluctant to address their concerns for fear that they will cause emotional pain for family members. Drawing a parallel to the new child is effective. If she were doing something hurtful to this child, would she not want her daughter or son to tell her so she could change it? This often overcomes any resistance about tackling these issues.

Group Therapy and Peer Support Groups. When available, peer support or therapy groups are an effective treatment for postpartum women. The strength of the peer-support movement in organizations such as Depression After Delivery and Postpartum Support International is an indication of the comfort and healing many women find in a group setting. Groups offer the woman a chance to heal by telling her story (Azar, 1994), and they provide immediate social support and validation. Clinical observations suggest that normalization and modeling effects are quite powerful. The limited research attesting to the success of such groups has been cited by Whiffen (1992) and Holden (1991).

Groups in the postpartum period take many forms. They can be process groups, led by trained therapists, or support groups facilitated by peers. Therapy groups may need to be closed, to prevent disruption of ongoing process, but peer-led groups are most often open. Groups can be time-limited and focused on specific topics, or open-ended and unstructured. Didactic groups focus on a topic each meeting, such as "anger" or "losses," and may invite professional speakers to address these topics. Clients with adjustment difficulties may prefer the structured, peer-led, open, and time-limited format; while clients with greater levels of distress and preexisting psychological dysfunction may need closed, ongoing, unstructured, process-type groups.

Gruen (1993) describes a structured, closed group in which phase-specific interventions are employed to educate women and their partners and decrease intensity and duration of symptoms. Phase I focuses on education and information, immediate stress reduction, and the beginning of cognitive restructuring and couple interventions. With phase II, symptoms decrease and the group focuses on continuing stress reduction, cognitive restructuring, and couple intervention, while adding a focus on rebuilding the new mother's self-esteem. Grief work is the focus of phase III, as the women come to terms with what having a postpartum disorder means and how to move forward. Gruen offers concrete interventions for each phase.

Clark et al. (1993) provide a detailed description of a group therapy model which includes the infant and the mother. Focus is on the mother's and the infant's individual needs, the mother-infant dyadic relationship, and the needs of spouse and family members. The group meets weekly for 12 weeks, for 2 hours, with a core theme each time such as depression, nurturance, or communication. The mothers are first separated from their infants and given a chance to receive support, validation, and nurturance. Infants are assigned a therapist to foster their development. The mother and child are reunited for dyadic activities, with a therapist guiding each dyad. Family members also interact with the therapist, receiving direction on communication, supporting the mother, and problem-solving.

Support groups are available in many parts of the United States, as well as Canada and other countries. Depression After Delivery and Postpartum Support International, listed on page 8, can identify groups in many parts of the country. They provide lists of telephone volunteers who will talk to new mothers if no group exists. These organizations offer advice and support for starting groups. If a group does not exist in the new mother's community, and starting one is not possible, the local mental health association may identify groups which educate or support parents. Religious organizations, postpartum exercise classes, and La Leche League or similar groups which support breast-feeding mothers may all be valuable. In some communities, play groups, baby-sitting cooperatives, and early childhood parent-teacher associations exist, providing networks of support for parents of young children. If no organized formats exist in a community, the family can find parents with children of similar ages and meet with those families regularly. Names of other families can be obtained from physician's offices or clergy.

The mother's partner is not to be neglected in support groups. Many support groups offer "dad's night"; therapy groups may also want to include the partner on a regular basis. Partners need this support as well, and should be encouraged to take advantage of the available resources.

PSYCHIATRIC INTERVENTION: MEDICATION AND HOSPITALIZATION

For many postpartum women, psychoactive medication is an important part of recovery. The new mother needs to be reassured that taking medication does not mean that she is weak or a failure. Rather, the need for medication suggests some chemical imbalance in her body which will resolve more quickly with the drug. Few medications are compatible with breast feeding. Only in mania and psychosis is medication absolutely essential for the new mother's health and the health of her baby. Contrary to widely accepted practice, obsessive thinking and panic symptoms do not require medication. Research and clinical experience have shown cognitive-behavioral interventions to be as effective with these conditions as medication. Postpartum women with these symptoms who wish to breast feed may be encouraged to do so.

In clinical practice, many postpartum women first talk to their obstetrician when seeking help. The obstetrician, as a medical professional, often sees medication as the first line of defense against postpartum distress. This quick tendency to bypass other therapeutic interventions can be especially unfortunate for the breast-feeding mother, because the prescribing of psychoactive drugs usually means a mother weans her baby. If she weans abruptly to take drugs, she may be setting herself back emotionally and biochemically as her hormones again need to achieve balance. Educating new families and health professionals about alternative treatments for postpartum distress is essential to temper this problem.

When is medication indicated for the postpartum woman? If she has been working diligently in therapy, and still does not feel better within 2 to 3 weeks, then medication may be needed. Preston and J. Johnson (1993) suggest that if a client is having significant difficulties with sleep disturbance, fatigue, restlessness/agitation, panic attacks, appetite changes, decreased sex drive, obsessive thoughts, mood variations throughout the day (especially worse in the morning), concentration difficulties/forgetfulness, lack of ability to feel pleasure, or psychotic symptoms, then psychoactive medication may be helpful. The therapist needs to weigh the normal symptoms of the postpartum period such as fatigue, concentration difficulties, and decreased sex drive against this list, especially for breast-feeding women. If the new mother's physical symptoms of depression, agitation, panic, or sleep disturbance are so powerful that she cannot follow through with the recommendations made in therapy, then a medication trial may be worthwhile. Bringing these symptoms to a manageable level, the mother will be able to continue her work in therapy.

Women with postpartum depression typically respond well to antidepressants, with about half of these women doing well on tricyclics while the other half seem to do best on selective serotonergic reuptake inhibitors (Wisner & Perel, 1991; Sichel, 1992). Current practice in treating postpartum women is toward multiple drug therapy, with a woman taking one medication for anxiety, an antidepressant, and often a medication for sleep. Combinations of antidepressants are not uncommon, with one antidepressant taken in the daytime and another taken at night to facilitate sleep. In clinical practice, lithium is also used frequently to augment the effect of an antidepressant. For refractory depressions, addition of lithium has been the turning point when the client finally begins to show real improvement.

Breast Feeding and Medications. Until recently, there was no debate about whether a breast-feeding woman could take psychoactive medications. The answer was a clear and resounding "No," due to the effect of the drug on the baby via the breast milk. Currently, most physicians still give this negative answer. Cohen (1992) and Wisner and associates (Wisner, Perel, & Foglia,1995; Wisner & Perel, 1991) have studied the levels of antidepressants in the breast milk and the baby's serum. While there are no blanket assurances, antidepressant medications which appear to be acceptable when a mother wishes to continue breast feeding are nortriptyline, imipramine, desipramine, sertraline, and clomipramine. Fluoxetine has produced mixed results. Carbamazepine (Tegretol) may be an acceptable medication for the postpartum woman with manic symptoms. Neuroleptics or antipsychotic medications may be used with breast-feeding mothers who suffer from mania or psychosis. According to the Marcé Society, these medications do enter the milk in small quantities, but there is no evidence in recent research that they affect the infant adversely. Information about antianxiety medication is sparse. The research that is available has indicated that lithium, diazepam, and doxepin are not compatible with breast feeding. This decision must be made on a case-by-case basis, with careful risk-benefit analysis. All of these researchers require that mothers who wish to take antidepressants and breast feed have regular lab evaluations of drug levels in both breast milk and the baby's serum. Caution is recommended; women should be alerted that there are no longitudinal studies following the children who have been exposed to medications in breast milk. Any long-term effects on the child's developing brain may not yet be evident, even with trace amounts of the drug in the breast milk. Newman (1994) presents a provocative argument, asserting that formula should be considered a drug. When evaluating breast milk with the possible effects of medication versus the effects of formula, he contends that formula is not a harmless choice. Research on formula-fed versus breast-fed babies indicates breast milk results in overall healthier babies.

Hormonal Interventions. There exists considerable controversy surrounding the use of hormones, particularly progesterone and estrogen, to treat postpartum disorders. Dalton (1985), the foremost proponent of using progesterone to treat postpartum depression, continues to feel it is immensely valuable (Dalton, 1993). Her claims about the value of this therapy have not been substantiated in double-blind, placebo-controlled trials (VanderMeer, Loendersloot, & VanLoenen, 1984). Many health professionals who work with postpartum women (Dunnewold & Sanford, 1994; Fernandez, 1992) report that progesterone therapy is beneficial for certain women. Recent research has shown that women who have a drastic fall in progesterone levels may be most at risk of depression (Harris et al., 1994; Steinberg, 1995). Use of progesterone does not jeopardize breast feeding, and may deserve consideration on a case-by-case basis. In clinical experience, there appear to be subtypes of postpartum women for whom progesterone therapy is most effective. Women with anxiety disorders, particularly panic and OCD with postpartum onset, seem to benefit well. Women with depressive symptoms may actually feel worse, especially if the depression dates to before or during pregnancy. Controlled research studies addressing the issue have not evaluated progesterone's effectiveness based on this kind of delineation of symptoms. If progesterone therapy is to be implemented, it must be started very quickly. The more days that pass postpartum, the less effective it may be. Dalton (1985) recommends beginning treatment at birth for best results; also natural progesterone, not synthetic, is used in her protocol.

Medical professionals have reported effective use of estrogen for treatment of postpartum disorders, particularly depression and psychosis (Sichel et al., 1995). Gregoire et al. (1996) detail a randomized, double-blind, placebo-controlled trial of therapy using estrogen skin patches. Further research is needed to identify the small subset of women who are most likely to respond well to this form of intervention.

Hospitalization. In some situations, hospitalization of the postpartum woman becomes necessary. This is most likely in postpartum psychosis or mania, but does occur in other cases if the new mother becomes suicidal. Suicide and homicide in this time period are rare, but the risk does arise with some postpartum women and needs quick, effective intervention. For a detailed discussion of the hospital care of the postpartum woman, see Sichel and Driscoll (1992).

In Great Britain, hospitalization of the new mother almost routinely includes the baby in order to avoid hindering the developing attachment. In the United States, designated mother-baby units are rare. In clinical experience, most private psychiatric facilities offer extensive visiting by the infant, so that the relationship with the baby is part of the treatment focus. Practitioners working with women should be aware of the critical necessity of including the baby on a daily basis in the mother's recovery, and be willing to become an advocate for the family to this end. If the new mother is so unstable that her interaction with the baby would put the baby at risk, plans should be made to postpone contact until she is stabilized. When mother-infant contact is resumed, support and guidance may be necessary to make that go smoothly.

The treatment that takes place while hospitalized takes the same path of education, reduction of symptoms, and focus on issues as does outpatient therapy (Sichel & Driscoll, 1992). When hospitalization becomes required, the guilt, shame, and loss of control that the new mother feels is usually heightened. All levels of medical caregivers must be extremely careful about making statements that will further fuel this guilt (Sichel & Driscoll, 1992). These feelings will require explicit intervention in order to avoid becoming a serious impediment to the therapy.

Electroconvulsive therapy (ECT) is an effective option with treatment-resistant patients (Sichel & Driscoll, 1992). These authors assert that the typical course of 6 to 12 treatments should not be prescribed, for often significant improvement is achieved with only 2 to 3 treatments. The idea of ECT usually further heightens the new mother's guilt, but careful discussion and education about this treatment can minimize these concerns. Emphasize that biochemical changes the new mother has undergone make ECT useful; this removes guilt because blame for the problems is attributed to physical, rather than psychological, causes.

INTEGRATING TREATMENT
APPROACHES: A CASE EXAMPLE

The care of the postpartum woman involves interdisciplinary cooperation and integration of individual, marital, group, and psychopharmacological therapies for effective treatment.

Vignette #3

Jan was a 31-year-old woman. She came for counseling when her son, Rob, was 4 months old. Jan had had two previous miscarriages. She and her husband had weathered those difficulties, and denied any marital distress. The pregnancy was normal; she was healthy and continued to work. Jan was breast feeding, and while she had a few blue days and some anxiety, the first 2 months were quite smooth.

Jan's symptoms began to develop at about 10 weeks postpartum after she and the baby visited with her parents at her girlhood home. When Jan and the baby had to return to their home, where her spouse was waiting, Jan began to get very anxious and upset. She did not want to go back, and was unable to tell her family why. She returned home, and promptly deteriorated. By the time the baby was 3 months old, Jan was not eating or drinking anything at all. She could not keep down solid food. She was unable to sleep, lying awake worrying about everything in her life. She was focusing on her marriage of 4 years. After 10 days of this, she went to stay with a married sister in another city, so that the sister could care for the baby while Jan "got some rest." Her husband supported this plan. In a week, Jan returned home, and then had a panic attack. Her husband took her to the emergency room; she was certain she would die. The physician on call prescribed an antidepressant and an antianxiety medication, and diagnosed her with postpartum depression. This was the first either Jan or her husband had considered the connection to the baby's birth, and it seemed to allow Jan to let go of the self-blame. She was able to find a therapist through the national network, Depression After Delivery.

In the first session, Jan was extremely upset. She cried almost nonstop, and would dissolve into near-hysteria as she worried about "the effect of this on my marriage." She was worried that she would never get better, and her husband would leave her. She stated that this was "all I ever wanted," and wondered how it could be turning out so poorly. She was unable to give much detail about why she feared for the marriage when she felt they had always been "so close." Flitting from topic to topic, Jan was distractible and forgetful. The initial session ended with only the immediate history gathered, for much of the time was spent on Jan expressing her feelings while the therapist validated them. The therapist assigned Jan homework to take care of herself each day. She still was not eating well, was throwing up frequently, and sleeping poorly. Arrangements were made for her to see a psychiatrist for medication. Over the next several sessions, Jan related her family history. She had a grandmother who committed suicide after a child's birth. Jan was very tied to her family-of-origin and talked to both her sisters and her mother daily via long distance. Jan described a normal upbringing, but was "mommy's baby girl" and had difficulty leaving home. Jan's previous adjustment had been problem-free; she had held a professional sales position. As Jan came to trust the therapist, her concerns about the marriage came out. Before the baby, Jan and her husband had been quite social, going to clubs, concerts, and drinking alcohol a great deal. After the baby's arrival, Jan's values had reverted to those of her family-of-origin, who frowned on consumption of alcohol. Immersed in the family again during that first visit home with Rob, Jan had begun to fear that her husband had a drinking problem. She was never sure when he would come home drunk, or at what hour. While she had tolerated this when she participated, it now felt like the end of the marriage, which would leave her as a single parent.

Given these concerns, a marital session was arranged. Jan canceled and rescheduled this session three times before she and her husband finally showed up. Contrary to the picture Jan had painted, her husband appeared reasonable and cooperative. She was extremely sensitive, and heard criticism from him in every sentence. Discussion centered openly on his drinking, which he denied was a problem, stating that he "liked to have a good time" and saw no reason to change his behavior. He presented all this in a rational manner; it was easy to see how Jan felt unnerved dealing with him at home. After this session, in which the couple resolved some religious differences, Jan was better for several weeks. The session left the therapist unsure of the state of the marriage. Jan was oversensitive and her husband may have been drinking to excess. Individual therapy continued with Jan, helping her grieve the separation from her family-of-origin, establish a network of social supports, and use behavioral techniques and journaling to decrease her anxiety.

Jan's progress was sporadic across the 5 months of therapy. She would do well for several weeks, then have a significant relapse, unable to eat. Then family contact increased, leading to Jan feeling better. Once, the psychiatrist switched her medication because Jan was unable to sleep. This helped briefly, and then Jan was off on this cycle again. Because of her unsteady progress, the therapist talked with Jan's primary-care physician, who completed in-depth thyroid studies, revealing no thyroid abnormalities. In therapy, Jan vacillated between calmly working on the issues, learning to take care of her emotional needs without relying on her family, and sobbing desperately about her life. She worked on asserting herself with her husband, and improving communication with him by asking him to clarify what he was saying whenever his comments made her feel attacked. Her husband attended marital sessions two more times, continuing to insist that Jan was oversensitive and that his drinking was not out of control. Jan attended a postpartum support group twice a month, which helped her recover hope that her life would improve. Jan was concerned about her relationship with the baby, so she brought him for several sessions of guidance on ways to improve their interaction. He was a thriving baby boy.

Because of this cycle of questionable progress, the therapist and psychiatrist set up a conjoint meeting with Jan and her husband, hoping to explore the marital relationship further. Before the meeting took place, Jan's husband was arrested for driving while intoxicated. Jan fell apart. In the session, she reported that she had been feeling suicidal for some time, and now was more so. The psychiatrist admitted Jan to the hospital. Her husband came for marital sessions three times weekly and a family group. In the supportive setting of the hospital, Jan confronted her husband about the drinking. With the pressures of his wife being hospitalized and his legal troubles, he began to open up. He admitted he was scared about being a parent, and feared duplicating his own family-of-origin with an alcoholic father. He agreed to get involved in Alcoholics Anonymous (AA), and Jan attended Alanon. During her stay, Jan had been switched to lithium from her antidepressants; this made a huge difference in her mood swings. After 10 days in the hospital, the picture for Jan and her family was brighter. Jan felt that her husband had hooked into the support system of AA, and even with work ahead, the family would survive. Jan continued her individual therapy, the support groups for postpartum moms, Alanon, and the marital therapy. By the time the baby was 10 months old, Jan was really able to enjoy having "all I ever wanted."

EARLY INTERVENTION
AND PREVENTION

In identifying women at risk for postpartum disorders, the practitioner needs to understand the influential factors described previously. Screening women for the presence of these risk factors during pregnancy, or before, is ideal. While there is not a standardized instrument for easily identifying women at risk, and efforts to develop one have been mixed (Appleby et al., 1994; C. T. Beck, 1995), having a working understanding of the salient factors is essential. Ideally, cooperation between primary care and mental health professionals would lead to education about, and assessment of, these issues with *all* women as they enter the childbearing years. At routine prepregnancy and prenatal visits, the system would have built-in checks for assessing a woman's mental health and the effect of pregnancy and postpartum. Women with increased risk would be monitored closely for symptom development during pregnancy. In the early postpartum period, the health professional would attend to the presence of sleeping difficulties, anxieties, and dysphoric mood. When care ends with the obstetrician or midwife, the responsibility for monitoring the mother's emotional state would be transferred to the child's physician, to be followed along with growth and development of the baby. In an ideal system, care like this would be standard. Assessment would be explicit, and accompanied by education and reassurance.

Continuing in this ideal system, women who had any risk factors would receive the next level of care. She would be offered support by knowledgeable, trained peers, and encouraged to establish a relationship with a mental health professional skilled in prenatal and/or postpartum issues. If unresolved issues needed to be addressed, this could be done during pregnancy, with an opportunity to rework those issues after the birth. Support during labor and birth could be provided; Wolman et al. (1993) found that such companionship and support greatly reduced rates of postpartum depression. If attention was paid to this process of emotional preparation for parenthood during pregnancy, many issues could be resolved and social support would be in place to take the mother through the postpartum period. Preliminary research shows that efforts to educate couples in this manner are successful (Coffman et al., 1994; Midmer, Wilson, & Cummings, 1995).

This ideal system is not in place in this country. Practitioners interested in postpartum issues can still help new families make these preparations. When meeting with parents-to-be, encourage them to evaluate their risk factors. Educate them about realistic expectations for postpartum adjustment; this can prevent guilt and feelings of failure when the time with a new baby seems less than wonderful. The therapist guides them through a plan for preventing or minimizing postpartum distress by applying the strategies for treatment described previously. Help them tackle the issues in their marital and extended family relationships, minimize the stresses in their lives by postponing major decisions in the childbearing year, and develop stress management skills and social supports that will carry them through this transition.

Community education is essential to advance the cause of early intervention and prevention. Many health professionals who work with pregnant women are eager to have this information. Childbirth educators, perinatal nurses, and midwives welcome speakers who can accurately address the emotional concerns of new parents. Research has shown that nurses tend to be more aware of aspects of postpartum depression than physicians, and within groups of physicians, younger, female physicians are more attuned to the disorder than older, male physicians (Lepper, DiMatteo, & Tinsley, 1994). In practical experience, this has been true; physicians often seem less interested in and educated about emotional outcomes. Perinatal professionals other than physicians have more contact with prenatal women, and provide valuable education on postpartum adjustment. Educational brochures and videos (see Dunnewold, 1995; Geyer & Gratz, 1995) on postpartum stress are effective tools in educating not only health professionals but prospective parents. Depression After Delivery and Postpartum Support International have brochures for this purpose, as does this author. Parent groups are very receptive to speakers with realistic information about postpartum emotions and are another valuable focus for community education.

The ultimate goal in prevention of postpartum distress is to incorporate a new view of motherhood into the culture. As Adcock (1993) states, images of motherhood can be constructed to incorporate reality rather than fantasy. Then women who find themselves experiencing negative emotions need no longer perceive themselves as failures. If society begins to recognize the difficult and demanding, but rewarding job of parenting as encompassing a range of feelings, women will no longer wonder "What is the matter with me?" They will find, instead, that their experience matches their expectations. Recognition of this reality will mean widespread support is readily available for the hard work and frustrations of parenting. This support can be a critical means of intervention for postpartum depression (LoCicero et al., 1995). As the anthropological literature makes clear (Kruckman, 1992), a supportive society can make all the difference in the life transition to parenthood.

SUMMARY

Cultural expectations and support for new mothers are slow to change. Given the widespread and continuing prevalence of postpartum emotional disorders, it is essential that mental health professionals understand these disorders and intervene effectively. A working knowledge of background and risk factors, the various symptom patterns, and the normal stresses inherent in this life transition are essential. Most importantly, however, therapists support and empower women to trust their own instincts and work to get their own needs met. New mothers need nurturing and coping skills; teaching and fostering these skills can provide not only a gratifying experience for the new mother in therapy but also a preventive mechanism for her continuing mental health and relationship with her child, partner, and family.

REFERENCES

Adcock, J. S. (1993). Expectations they cannot meet: Understanding postnatal depression. *Professional Nurse, 8,* 703-
710.

Affonso, D. D., & Arizmendi, T. G. (1986). Disturbances in
postpartum adaptation and depressive symptomatology. *Journal of Psychosomatic Obstetrics and Gynecology, 5,* 15-
32.

Affonso, D. D., Lovett, S., Paul, S. M., & Sheptak, S. (1990).
A standardized interview that differentiates pregnancy and postpartum symptoms from perinatal clinical depression. *Birth,
17,* 121-130.

Affonso, D. D., Lovett, S., Paul, S., Sheptak, S., Nussbaum, R.,
Newman, L., & Johnson, B. (1992). Dysphoric distress in
child-bearing women. *Journal of Perinatalogy, 12,* 325-332.

American Psychiatric Association. (1952). *Diagnostic and Statistical Manual of Mental Disorders (DSM).* Washington,
DC: Author.

American Psychiatric Association. (1994). *Diagnostic and Statistical Manual of Mental Disorders (DSM-IV).* Washington, DC: Author.

Appleby, L., Gregoire, A., Platz, C., Prince, M., & Kumar, R.
(1994). Screening women for high risk of postnatal depression. *Journal of Psychosomatic Research, 38,* 539-545.

Arizmendi, T. G., & Affonso, D. D. (1987). Stressful events related to pregnancy and postpartum. *Journal of Psychosomatic Research, 31,* 743-756.

Arts, W., Hoogduin, K., Schaap, C., & de Haan, E. (1993). Do patients suffering from obsessions alone differ from other obsessive-compulsives? *Behavior Research and Therapy, 31,* 119-123.

Atkinson, A. K., & Rickel, A. U. (1984). Postpartum depression in primiparous parents. *Journal of Abnormal Psychology, 93,* 115-119.

Azar, B. (1994, November). Research plumbs why the "talking cure" works. *APA Monitor,* p. 24.

Ballard, C. G., Davis, R., Cullen, P. C., Mohan, R. N., & Dean, C. (1994). Prevalence of postnatal psychiatric morbidity in mothers and fathers. *British Journal of Psychiatry, 164,* 782-788.

Barnett, B., & Parker, G. (1985). Professional and nonprofessional intervention for highly anxious primiparous mothers. *British Journal of Psychiatry, 146,* 287-293.

Bebbington, P. E., Dean, C., Der, G., Hurry, J., & Tennant, C. (1991). Gender, parity, and the prevalence of minor affective disorder. *British Journal of Psychiatry, 158,* 40-45.

Beck, A. T., Ward, C. H., Mendelson, M., Mock, J. E., & Erbaugh, J. K. (1961). An inventory for measuring depression. *Archives of General Psychiatry, 4,* 561-569.

Beck, C. T. (1995). Screening methods for postpartum depression. *Journal of Obstetric, Gynecologic, and Neonatal Nursing, 24,* 308-312.

Bennett, D. E., & Slade, P. (1991). Infants born at risk: Consequences for maternal postpartum adjustment. *British Journal of Medical Psychology, 64*(2), 159-172.

Bonnin, F. (1992). Cortisol levels in saliva and mood changes in early puerperium. *Journal of Affective Disorders, 26,* 231-240.

Bourne, E. J. (1990). *The Anxiety and Phobia Workbook.* Oakland, CA: New Harbinger Publications.

Brockington, I. F., & Cox-Roper, A. (1988). The nosology of puerperal mental illness. In R. Kumar & I. F. Brockington (Eds.), *Motherhood and Mental Illness 2: Causes and Consequences* (pp. 1-16). London: Butterworth & Co. Ltd.

Bruce, M., Scott, N., Shine, P., & Lader, M. (1992). Anxiogenic effects of caffeine in patients with anxiety disorders. *Archives of General Psychiatry, 49,* 867-869.

Burger, J., Horwitz, S. M., Forsyth, B., Leventhal, J. M., & Leaf, P. J. (1993). Psychological sequelae of medical complications during pregnancy. *Pediatrics, 91,* 566-572.

Campbell, S. B., & Cohn, J. F. (1991). Prevalence and correlates of postpartum depression in first-time mothers. *Journal of Abnormal Psychology, 100,* 594-599.

Campbell, S. B., Cohn, J. F., Flanagan, C., Popper, S., & Meyers, T. (1992). Course and correlates of postpartum depression during the transition to parenthood. *Development and Psychopathology, 4,* 29-47.

Chrousos, G. P. (1995). Hypothalamic corticotropin-releasing hormone suppression during the postpartum period: Implications for the increase of psychiatric manifestations in this period. *Science News, 148,* 260-270.

Clark, R., Keller, A. D., Fedderly, S. S., & Paulson, A. W. (1993). Treating the relationships affected by postpartum depression: A group therapy model. *Zero to Three, 13*(5), 16-23.

Clum, G. A., & Surls, R. (1993). A meta-analysis of treatments for panic disorder. *Journal of Consulting and Clinical Psychology, 61,* 317-236.

Coffman, S., Levitt, M. J., & Brown, L. (1994). Effects of clarification of support expectations in prenatal couples. *Nursing Research, 43,* 111-116.

Cohen, L. S. (1992). The use of psychotropic drugs during pregnancy and the puerperium. *Currents in Affective Illness, 11*(9), 5-13.

Collins, N. L., Dunkel-Schetter, C., Lobel, M., & Scrimshaw, S. (1993). Psychosocial correlates of birth outcomes and postpartum depression. *Journal of Personality and Social Psychology, 65,* 1243-1258.

Cooper, P. J., Campbell, E. A., Day, A., Kennerley, H., & Bond, A. (1988). Non-psychotic psychiatric disorder after childbirth: A prospective study of prevalence, incidence, course, and nature. *British Journal of Psychiatry, 152,* 799-806.

Cowan, C. P., & Cowan, P. A. (1987). A preventive intervention for couples becoming parents. In C. F. Z. Boukydis (Ed.), *Research on Support for Parents and Infants in the Postnatal Period* (pp. 225-252). Norwood, NJ: Ablex.

Cox, J. L., Holden, J. M., & Sagovsky, R. (1987). Detection of postnatal depression: Development of the ten-item Edinburgh Postnatal Depression Scale. *British Journal of Psychiatry, 150,* 782-786.

Cox, J. L., Murray, D., & Chapman, G. (1993). A controlled study of the onset, duration, and prevalence of postnatal depression. *British Journal of Psychiatry, 163,* 27-31.

Cramer, B. (1993). Are postpartum depressions a mother-infant relationship disorder? *Infant Mental Health Journal, 14,* 283-297.

Cutrona, C. (1984). Social support and stress in the transition to parenthood. *Journal of Abnormal Psychology, 93,* 378-390.

Cutrona, C., & Troutman, B. R. (1986). Social support, infant temperament, and parenting self-efficacy: A mediational model of postpartum depression. *Child Development, 57,* 1507-1518.

Dalton, K. (1985). Progesterone prophylaxis used successfully in postnatal depression. *The Practitioner: The Journal of Postgraduate Medicine, 229,* 507-508.

Dalton, K. (1993, June). *Prophylactic Progesterone for Postnatal Depression.* Paper presented at the annual meeting of Postpartum Support International, Chicago, IL.

Davis, J. C., & Abou-Saleh, M. T. (1992). Psychiatric manifestations in patients with postpartum hypopituitarism. In J. A. Hamilton & P. N. Harberger (Eds.), *Postpartum Psychiatric*

Illness: A Picture Puzzle (pp. 191-199). Philadelphia: University of Pennsylvania Press.

Demyttenaere, K., Lenaerts, H., Nijs, P., & Van Assche, F. A. (1995). Individual coping style and psychological attitudes during pregnancy predict depression levels during pregnancy and during postpartum. *Acta Psychiatrica Scandinavica, 91,* 95-102.

Dix, C. (1985). *The New Mother Syndrome.* New York: Pocket.

Donovan, W. L., & Leavitt, L. A. (1989). Maternal self-efficacy and infant attachment: Integrating physiology, perceptions, and behavior. *Child Development, 60,* 460-472.

Donovan, W. L., Leavitt, L. A., & Walsh, R. O. (1990). Maternal self-efficacy: Illusory control and its effect on susceptibility to learned helplessness. *Child Development, 61,* 1638-1647.

Downey, G., & Coyne, J. C. (1990). Children of depressed parents: An integrative review. *Psychological Bulletin, 108,* 50-76.

Dunnewold, A. (1995). *Postpartum Stress.* (Brochure available from Postpartum Wellness Resources, P.O. Box 742094, Dallas, TX 75374-2094.)

Dunnewold, A., & Sanford, D. (1994). *Postpartum Survival Guide.* Oakland, CA: New Harbinger Publications.

Edwards, D. R. L., Porter, S. M., & Stein, G. S. (1994). A pilot study of postnatal depression following Caesarean section using two retrospective self-rating instruments. *Journal of Psychosomatic Research, 38,* 111-117.

Endicott, J., & Spitzer, R. (1978). A diagnostic interview for affective disorders and schizophrenia. *Archives of General Psychiatry, 35,* 837-844.

Feggetter, P., & Gath, D. (1981). Nonpsychotic psychiatric disorders in women one year after childbirth. *Journal of Psychosomatic Research, 25,* 369-372.

Fernandez, R. (1992). Recent clinical management experience. In J. A. Hamilton & P. N. Harberger (Eds.), *Postpartum Psychiatric Illness: A Picture Puzzle* (pp. 78-89). Philadelphia: University of Pennsylvania Press.

Field, T. (1987). Interaction and attachment in normal and atypical infants. *Journal of Consulting and Clinical Psychology, 55,* 853-859.

Field, T., Healy, B., Goldstein, S., & Guthertz, M. (1990). Behavior-state matching and synchrony in mother-infant interactions of nondepressed versus depressed dyads. *Developmental Psychology, 26,* 7-14.

Field, T., Morrow, C., Healy, B., Foster, T., Adelstein, D., & Goldstein, S. (1991). Mothers with zero Beck Depression scores act more depressed with their infants. *Development and Psychopathology, 3,* 253-262.

Filer, R. B. (1992). Endocrinology in the postpartum period. In J. A. Hamilton & P. N. Harberger (Eds.), *Postpartum Psychiatric Illness: A Picture Puzzle* (pp. 153-163). Philadelphia: University of Pennsylvania Press.

Foa, E. (1992). *Behavioral Treatment of Obsessive-Compulsive Disorder.* Training institute conducted at the annual meeting of the Anxiety Disorders Association of America, Houston, TX.

Ford, G. (1992). *What's Wrong With My Hormones?* Newcastle, CA: Desmond Ford Publications.

Frommer, E. A., & O'Shea, G. (1973). Antenatal identification of women liable to have problems in managing their infants. *British Journal of Psychiatry, 123,* 149-156.

Geyer, R. A., Jr. (Producer), & Gratz, V. (Director). (1995). Postpartum Emotions: The Blues and Beyond [Videotape]. (Available from Family Experience Productions, Inc., P.O. Box 5879, Austin, TX 78763-5879; 512-494-0338)

Gitlin, M. J., & Pasnau, R. O. (1989). Psychiatric syndromes linked to reproductive function in women: A review of current knowledge. *American Journal of Psychiatry, 146,* 1413-1422.

Gjerdingen, D. K., & Chaloner, K. M. (1994). The relationship of women's postpartum mental health to employment, childbirth, and social support. *Journal of Family Practice, 38,* 465-473.

Gjerdingen, D. K., Froberg, D. G., Chaloner, K. M., & McGovern, P. M. (1993). Changes in women's physical health during the first postpartum year. *Archives of Family Medicine, 2,* 277-283.

Gordon, R. E., & Gordon, K. K. (1959). Social factors in the prediction and treatment of emotional disorders of pregnancy. *American Journal of Obstetrics and Gynecology, 77,* 1074-1083.

Gotlib, I. H., Whiffen, V. E., Mount, J. H., Milne, K., & Cordy, N. I. (1989). Prevalence rates and demographic characteristics associated with depression in pregnancy and the postpartum. *Journal of Consulting and Clinical Psychology, 57,* 269-274.

Gotlib, I. H., Whiffen, V. E., Wallace, P. M., & Mount, J. H. (1991). Prospective investigation of postpartum depression: Factors involved in onset and recovery. *Journal of Abnormal Psychology, 100,* 122-132.

Gottman, J. M. (1993). *What Predicts Divorce? The Relationship Between Marital Processes and Marital Outcomes.* Hillsdale, NJ: Erlbaum.

Greenberg, M. (1985). *The Birth of a Father.* New York: Avon Books.

Gregoire, A. J. P., Kumar, R., Everitt, B., Henderson, A. F., & Studd, J. W. W. (1996). Transdermal oestrogen for treatment of severe postnatal depression. *The Lancet, 347,* 930-933.

Gruen, D. S. (1993). A group psychotherapy approach to postpartum depression. *International Journal of Group Psychotherapy, 43,* 191-203.

Haggerty, J. J., Jr., Stern, R. A., Mason, G. A., Beckwith, J., Morey, C. E., Prange, A. J., Jr. (1993). Subclinical hypothyroidism: A modifiable risk factor for depression? *American Journal of Psychiatry, 150,* 508-510.

Halonen, J. S., & Passman, R. H. (1985). Relaxation training and expectation in the treatment of postpartum distress. *Journal of Consulting and Clinical Psychology, 53,* 839-845.

Hamilton, J. M. (1992). Patterns of postpartum illness. In J. A. Hamilton & P. N. Harberger (Eds.), *Postpartum Psychiatric Illness: A Picture Puzzle* (pp. 5-14). Philadelphia: University of Pennsylvania Press.

Hamilton, J. M., & Sichel, D. A. (1992). Prophylactic measures. In J. A. Hamilton & P. N. Harberger (Eds.), *Postpartum Psychiatric Illness: A Picture Puzzle* (pp. 219-234). Philadelphia: University of Pennsylvania Press.

Handley, S. L., Dunn, T. L., Baker, J. M., Cockshott, C., & Gould, S. (1977). Mood changes in puerperium, and plasma tryptophan and cortisol concentrations. *British Medical Journal, 2,* 18-22.

Handley, S. L., Dunn, T. L., Waldron, G., & Baker, J. M. (1980). Tryptophan, cortisol, and puerperal mood. *British Journal of Psychiatry, 136,* 498-508.

Hannah, P., Adams, D., Lee, A., Glover, V., & Sandler, M. (1992). Links between early postpartum mood and postnatal depression. *British Journal of Psychiatry, 160,* 777-780.

Harris, B., Johns, S., Fung, H., Thomas, R., Walker, R., Read, G., & Riad-Fahmy, D. (1989). The hormonal environment of postnatal depression. *British Journal of Psychiatry, 154,* 660-667.

Harris, B., Lovett, L., Newcombe, R. G., Read, G. F., Walker, R., & Riad-Fahmy, D. (1994). Maternity blues and major endocrine changes: Cardiff puerperal mood and hormone study II. *British Medical Journal, 308,* 949-955.

Harris, B., Othman, S., Davies, J. A., Weppner, G. J., Richards, C. J., Newcombe, R. G., Lazarus, J. H., Parkes, A. B., Hall, R., & Phillips, D. I. W. (1992). Association between postpartum thyroid dysfunction and thyroid antibodies and depression. *British Medical Journal, 305*(5), 152-157.

Hickman, S. (1994, June). *What About the Children?* Presentation at the annual meeting of Postpartum Support International, Toronto, Canada.

Hobfoll, S. E., Ritter, C., Lavin, J., Hulsizer, M. R., & Cameron, R. P. (1995). Depression prevalence and incidence among inner-city pregnant and postpartum women. *Journal of Consulting and Clinical Psychology, 63,* 445-453.

Holden, J. M. (1991). Postnatal depression: Its nature, effects, and identification using the Edinburgh Postnatal Depression Scale. *Birth, 18,* 211-223.

Hopkins, J., Campbell, S. B., & Marcus, M. (1987). Role of infant-related stressors in postpartum depression. *Journal of Abnormal Psychology, 96,* 237-241.

Hopkins, J., Campbell, S. B., & Marcus, M. (1989). Postpartum depression and postpartum adaptation: Overlapping constructs? *Journal of Affective Disorders, 17,* 251-254.

Hopkins, J., Marcus, M., & Campbell, S. B. (1984). Postpartum depression: A critical review. *Psychological Bulletin, 95,* 498-515.

Iles, S., Gath, D., & Kennerley, H. (1989). Maternity blues: II. A comparison between post-operative women and postnatal women. *British Journal of Psychiatry, 155,* 363-366.

Joyce, P. R., Rogers, J. R., & Anderson, E. D. (1981). Mania associated with weaning. *British Journal of Psychiatry, 139,* 355-356.

Kalmuss, D., Davidson, A., & Cushman, L. (1992). Expectations and experience of parenthood. *Journal of Marriage and the Family, 54,* 516-526.

Kendall-Tackett, K. A., & Kantor, G. K. (1993). *Postpartum Depression: A Comprehensive Approach for Nurses.* Newbury Park, CA: Sage.

Klerman, G. L., Weissman, M. M., Rounsaville, B. J., & Chevron, E. S. (1984). *Interpersonal Psychotherapy of Depression.* New York: Basic Books.

Knops, G. G. (1993). Postpartum mood disorders: A startling contrast to the joy of birth. *Postgraduate Medicine, 93*(3), 103-116.

Krause, M. A., & Redman, E. S. (1986). Postpartum depression: An interactional view. *Journal of Marital and Family Therapy, 12,* 63-74.

Kruckman, L. D. (1992). Rituals and support: An anthropological view of postpartum depression. In J. A. Hamilton & P. N. Harberger (Eds.), *Postpartum Psychiatric Illness: A Picture Puzzle* (pp. 137-148). Philadelphia: University of Pennsylvania Press.

Kumar, R., & Robson, K. M. (1984). A prospective study of emotional disorders in childbearing women. *British Journal of Psychiatry, 144,* 35-47.

Lansky, V. (Ed.). (1993). *Games Babies Play: From Birth to Twelve Months.* Deephaven, MN: The Book Peddlers.

Lepper, H. S., DiMatteo, M. R., & Tinsley, B. J. (1994). Postpartum depression: How much do obstetric nurses and obstetricians know? *Birth, 21,* 149-154.

Levy, V. (1987). The maternity blues in postpartum and postoperative women. *British Journal of Psychiatry, 151,* 368-372.

LoCicero, A. K., Weiss, D., & Issokson, D. (1995, August). *Postpartum Depression: Promising Preventive Interventions Consistent With Social Science Research.* Paper presented at the annual convention of the American Psychological Association, New York City, NY.

Markman, H., & Notarius, C. (1994). *Fighting for Your Marriage: Preventing Divorce and Preserving a Lasting Love.* San Francisco: Jossey-Bass.

McGrath, E. (1992). *When Feeling Bad Is Good.* New York: Henry Holt and Co.

McKay, M. (Producer), & Mitchell, G. (Director). (1995). *Couple Skills* [Videotape]. (Available from New Harbinger Publications, Inc., 5674 Shattuck Avenue, Oakland, CA 94609)

McKay, M., Fanning, P., & Paleg, K. (1994). *Couple Skills.* Oakland, CA: New Harbinger Publications.

Metz, A., Sichel, D. A., & Goff, D. C. (1988). Postpartum panic disorder. *Journal of Clinical Psychiatry, 49,* 278-279.

Midmer, D., Wilson, L., & Cummings, S. (1995). A randomized, controlled trial of the influence of prenatal parenting education on postpartum anxiety and marital adjustment. *Family Medicine, 27*(3), 200-205.

Miller, A. R., Barr, R. G., & Eaton, W. O. (1993). Crying and motor behavior of six-week-old infants and postpartum maternal mood. *Pediatrics, 92,* 551-559.

Moleman, N., Van der Hart, O., & Van der Kolk, B. A. (1992). The partus stress reaction: A neglected etiological factor in postpartum psychiatric disorders. *Journal of Nervous and Mental Disease, 180,* 271-272.

Morin, C. M., Stone, J., McDonald, K., & Jones, S. (1994). Psychological management of insomnia: A clinical replication series with 100 patients. *Behavior Therapy, 25,* 291-309.

Munger, E. M., & Bowden, S. J. (1993). *The New Beyond Peek-A-Boo and Pattycake: Activities for Baby's First Twenty-Four Months.* Piscataway, NJ: New Century Publishers.

Murray, L., Cooper, P. J., & Stein, A. (1991). Postnatal depression and infant development. *British Medical Journal, 302,* 978-980.

Newman, J. (1994, June). *A Postpartum Mood and Anxiety Disorder Diagnosis and Breastfeeding: Facts, Fiction, and Feelings.* Presentation at the annual conference of Postpartum Support International, Toronto, Ontario, Canada.

Neziroglu, F., Anemone, R., & Yaryura-Tobias, J. A. (1992). Onset of obsessive-compulsive disorder in pregnancy. *American Journal of Psychiatry, 149,* 947-950.

Nomura, J., & Okano, T. (1992). Endocrine function and hormonal treatment of postpartum psychosis. In J. A. Hamilton & P. N. Harberger (Eds.), *Postpartum Psychiatric Illness: A Picture Puzzle* (pp. 176-190). Philadelphia: University of Pennsylvania Press.

O'Hara, M. W. (1986). Social support, life events, and depression during pregnancy and the puerperium. *Archives of General Psychiatry, 43,* 596-573.

O'Hara, M. W. (1996, September). *Interpersonal Psychotherapy for Postpartum Depression: Preliminary Findings.*

Paper presented at the biennial meeting of the Marcé Society, London, England.

O'Hara, M. W., Hoffman, J. G., Philipps, L. H. C., & Wright, E. J. (1992). Adjustment in childbearing women: The Postpartum Adjustment Questionnaire. *Psychological Assessment, 4,* 160-169.

O'Hara, M. W., Neunaber, D. J., & Zekoski, E. M. (1984). A prospective study of postpartum depression: Prevalence, course, and predictive factors. *Journal of Abnormal Psychology, 93,* 158-171.

O'Hara, M. W., Rehm, L. P., & Campbell, S. B. (1982). Predicting depressive symptomatology: Cognitive-behavioral models and postpartum depression. *Journal of Abnormal Psychology, 91,* 457-461.

O'Hara, M. W., Rehm, L. P., & Campbell, S. B. (1983). Postpartum depression: A role for social network and life stress variables. *Journal of Nervous and Mental Disease, 171,* 336-341.

O'Hara, M. W., Schlechte, J. A., Lewis, D. A., & Varner, M. W. (1991). Controlled prospective study of postpartum mood disorders: Psychological, environmental, and hormonal variables. *Journal of Abnormal Psychology,* 100, 63-73.

O'Hara, M. W., Schlechte, J. A., Lewis, D. A., & Wright, E. J. (1991). Prospective study of postpartum blues: Biologic and psychosocial factors. *Archives of General Psychiatry, 48,* 801-806.

O'Hara, M. W., & Zekoski, E. M. (1988). Postpartum depression: A comprehensive review. In R. Kumar & I. F. Brockington (Eds.), *Motherhood and Mental Illness 2: Causes and Consequences* (pp. 17-63). London: Butterworth & Co. Ltd.

O'Hara, M. W., Zekoski, E. M., Philipps, L. H., & Wright, E. J. (1990). Controlled prospective study of postpartum mood disorders: Comparison of childbearing and nonchildbearing women. *Journal of Abnormal Psychology, 99,* 3-15.

Parker, S. J., & Barrett, D. E. (1992). Maternal type A behavior during pregnancy, neonatal crying, and early infant temperament: Do type A women have type A babies? *Pediatrics, 89,* 474-479.

Parry, B. L., (1992). Reproductive-related depressions in women: Phenomenon of hormone kindling? In J. A. Hamilton & P. N. Harberger (Eds.), *Postpartum Psychiatric Illness: A Picture Puzzle* (pp. 200-218). Philadelphia: University of Pennsylvania Press.

Paykel, E. S., Emms, E. M., Fletcher, J., & Rassaby, E. S. (1980). Life events and social support in puerperal depression. *British Journal of Psychiatry, 136,* 339-346.

Pearlstein, T. (1993, June). *Diagnosing and Treating Late Luteal Phase Dysphoric Disorder.* Presentation at the conference on Psychiatric Disorders Associated With Female Reproductive Function, Harvard Medical School, Boston, MA.

Pfost, K. S., Stevens, M. J., & Lum, C. U. (1990). The relationship of demographic variables, antepartum depression, and stress to postpartum depression. *Journal of Clinical Psychology*, 46, 588-592.

Philipps, L. H. C., & O'Hara, M. W. (1991). Prospective study of postpartum depression: 4.5 year follow-up of women and children. *Journal of Abnormal Psychology, 100,* 151-156.

Pickens, J., & Field, T. (1993). Attention-getting vs. imitation effects on depressed mother-infant interactions. *Infant Mental Health Journal, 14,* 171-181.

Pitt, B. (1968). "Atypical" depression following childbirth. *British Journal of Psychiatry*, 114, 1325-1335.

Pop, V. J. M., Essed, G. G. M., De Geus, C. A., Van Son, M. M., & Komproe, I. H. (1993). Prevalence of post partum depression - or is it post-puerperium depression? *Acta Obstetricia et Gynecologica Scandinavica, 72,* 354-358.

Preston, J., & Johnson, J. (1993). *Clinical Psychopharmocology Made Ridiculously Simple.* Miami: MedMaster, Inc.

Roemer, L., & Borkovec, T. D. (1994). Effects of suppressing thoughts about emotional material. *Journal of Abnormal Psychology, 103*, 467-474.

Rohde, A., & Marneros, A. (1993). Postpartum psychoses: Onset and long-term course. *Psychopathology, 26*, 203-209.

Roth, A. D., & Church, J. A. (1994). The use of revised habituation in the treatment of obsessive-compulsive disorders. *British Journal of Clinical Psychology, 33*, 201-204.

Salkovskis, P. M., & Campbell, P. (1994). Thought suppression induces intrusion in naturally occurring negative intrusive thoughts. *Behavior Research and Therapy, 32*, 1-8.

Sholomskas, D. E., Wickamaratne, P. J., Dogolo, L., O'Brien, D. W., Leaf, P. J., & Woods, S. W. (1993). *Journal of Clinical Psychiatry, 54*, 476-480.

Sichel, D. A. (1990, June). *Current Research.* Paper presented at the annual meeting of Postpartum Support International, St. Louis, MO.

Sichel, D. A. (1992). Psychiatric issues of the postpartum period. *Currents in Affective Illness, 11*(10), 5-12.

Sichel, D. A., Cohen, L. S., Dimmock, J. A., & Rosenbaum, J. F. (1993). Postpartum obsessive compulsive disorder: A case series. *Journal of Clinical Psychiatry, 54*, 156-159.

Sichel, D. A., Cohen, L. S., Robertson, L. M., Ruttenberg, A., & Rosenbaum, J. (1995). Prophylactic estrogen in recurrent postpartum affective disorders. *Biological Psychiatry, 38*, 814-818.

Sichel, D. A., & Driscoll, J. W. (1992). The integrated care of hospitalized women with postpartum psychiatric illness. In J. A. Hamilton & P. N. Harberger (Eds.), *Postpartum Psychiatric Illness: A Picture Puzzle* (pp. 115-125). Philadelphia: University of Pennsylvania Press.

Slade, P., MacPherson, S. A., Hume, A., & Maresh, M. (1993). Expectations, experiences, and satisfaction with labour. *British Journal of Clinical Psychology, 32*, 469-483.

Smith, R., & Singh, B. (1992). The hypothalamic-pituitary-adrenal axis and mood disorders related to pregnancy. In J. A.

Hamilton & P. N. Harberger (Eds.), *Postpartum Psychiatric Illness: A Picture Puzzle* (pp. 164-175). Philadelphia: University of Pennsylvania Press.

Spitzer, R., Endicott, J., & Robins, E. (1981). *Research Diagnostic Criteria (RDQ)* (1st ed.). New York: New York Psychiatric Institute, Biometrics Research.

Stein, G., & Van den Akker, O. (1992). The retrospective diagnosis of postnatal depression by questionnaire. *Journal of Psychosomatic Research, 36,* 67-75.

Steinberg, S. (1995, April). *Progesterone Metabolites: Their Relationship to Depression During Pregnancy.* Paper presented at Marcé Society Pacific Rim Conference, Sydney, Australia.

Stern, E. S. (1986). *Expecting Change: The Emotional Journey Through Pregnancy.* New York: Poseidon.

Stevenson-Hinde, J. (1990). Attachment in family systems: An overview. *Infant Mental Health Journal, 11,* 218-227.

Stuart, S., & O'Hara, M. W. (1995). Treatment of postpartum depression with interpersonal psychotherapy. *Archives of General Psychiatry, 52,* 75-76.

Susman, V. L., & Katz, J. L. (1988). Weaning and depression: Another postpartum complication. *American Journal of Psychiatry, 145,* 498-501.

Tallis, F. (1993). Primary hypothyroidism: A case of vigilance in the psychological treatment of depression. *British Journal of Clinical Psychology, 32,* 261-270.

VanderMeer, Y. G., Loendersloot, E. W., & VanLoenen, A. C. (1984). Effect of high-dose progesterone in postpartum depression. *Journal of Psychosomatic Obstetrics and Gynecology, 3,* 67-68.

Van Oppen, P., & Arntz, A. (1994). Cognitive therapy for obsessive-compulsive disorder. *Behavior Research and Therapy, 32,* 79-87.

Watson, E., & Evans, S. J. (1986). An example of cross-cultural measurement of psychological symptoms in postpartum mothers. *Social Science and Medicine, 23,* 869-874.

Watson, J. P., Elliot, S. A., Rugg, A. J., & Brough, D. I. (1984). Psychiatric disorder in pregnancy and the first postnatal year. *British Journal of Psychiatry, 144*, 453-462.

Watts, F. N., Coyle, K., & East, M. P. (1994). The contribution of worry to insomnia. *British Journal of Clinical Psychology, 33*, 211-220.

Whiffen, V. E. (1988). Vulnerability to postpartum depression: A prospective, multivariate study. *Journal of Abnormal Psychology, 97*, 467-474.

Whiffen, V. E. (1992). Is postpartum depression a distinct diagnosis? *Clinical Psychology Review, 12*, 498-508.

Whiffen, V. E., & Gotlib, I. H. (1993). Comparison of postpartum and nonpostpartum depression: Clinical presentation, psychiatric history, and psychosocial functioning. *Journal of Consulting and Clinical Psychology, 61*, 485-494.

Wilkie, G., & Shapiro, C. M. (1992). Sleep deprivation and the postnatal blues. *Journal of Psychosomatic Research, 36*, 309-316.

Wilson, R. R. (1986). *Don't Panic: Taking Control of Anxiety Attacks.* New York: Harper Perennial.

Wisner, K. L., & Perel, J. M. (1991). Serum nortriptyline levels in nursing mothers and their infants. *American Journal of Psychiatry, 148*, 1234-1236.

Wisner, K. L., Perel, J. M., & Foglia, J. P. (1995). Serum clomipramine and metabolite levels in four nursing mother-infant pairs. *Journal of Clinical Psychiatry, 56*, 17-20.

Wohlreich, M. M. (1994). Postpartum emotional illness: Recognition and management in primary care. *Journal of the South Carolina Medical Association, 90*, 120-127.

Wolman, W. L., Chalmers, B., Hofmeyr, G. J., & Nikodem, C. (1993). Postpartum depression and companionship in the clinical birth environment: A randomized, controlled study. *American Journal of Obstetrics and Gynecology, 168*, 1388-1394.

World Health Organization. (1978). *Mental Disorders: Glossary and Guide to the Classification in Accordance With the 9th Revision of the International Classification of Disease (ICD-9)*. Geneva: Author.

York, R., Volpicelli, J., Brooten, D., Charche, D., & Speicher, M. (1992). Mood disturbances during pregnancy and postpartum depression. *The Journal of Perinatal Education, 1*(3), 13-20.

Zekoski, E. M., O'Hara, M. W., & Wills, K. E. (1987). The effects of maternal mood on mother-infant interaction. *Journal of Abnormal Child Psychology, 15,* 361-378.